Handbook of
Pulmonary
Emergencies

Handbook of
Pulmonary
Emergencies

Edited by

Samuel V. Spagnolo, M.D., F.A.C.P., F.C.C.P.

Professor of Medicine
Director, Division of Pulmonary Diseases and Allergy
and Associate Chairman, Department of Medicine
George Washington School of Medicine and Health Sciences
and Chief, Pulmonary Disease Section
Veterans Administration Medical Center
Washington, D.C.

and

Ann Medinger, M.D., F.A.C.P., F.C.C.P.

Assistant Professor of Medicine
Division of Pulmonary Diseases and Allergy
George Washington School of Medicine and Health Sciences
and Chief, Pulmonary Function Laboratory
Veterans Administration Medical Center
Washington, D.C.

Plenum Medical Book Company
New York and London

Library of Congress Cataloging in Publication Data

Handbook of pulmonary emergencies.

Includes bibliographies and index.
1. Lungs — Diseases — Handbooks, manuals, etc. 2. Medical emergencies — Handbooks, manuals, etc. I. Spagnolo, Samuel V. II. Medinger, Ann. [DNLM; 1. Emergencies. 2. Lung Diseases — therapy. QF 140 H2377]
RC756.H29   1986   616.2′00425   86-15064
ISBN-13: 978-1-4684-5127-6   e-ISBN-13: 978-1-4684-5125-2
DOI: 10.1007/978-1-4684-5125-2

© 1986 Plenum Publishing Corporation
233 Spring Street, New York, N.Y. 10013
Softcover reprint of the hardcover 1st edition 1986

Plenum Medical Book Company is an imprint of Plenum Publishing Corporation

Contributors

Aram A. Arabian, M.D., Assistant Professor of Medicine, Division of Pulmonary Diseases and Allergy, George Washington University School of Medicine and Health Sciences, Washington, D.C. 20037; Chief, Respiratory Care, Veterans Administration Medical Center, Washington, D.C. 20422

Morgan D. Delaney, M.D., Associate Professor of Medicine, Director, Pulmonary Laboratory, Division of Pulmonary Diseases and Allergy, George Washington University School of Medicine and Health Sciences, Washington, D.C. 20037

Kenneth Dickie, M.D., Associate Professor of Medicine, Division of Pulmonary Diseases and Allergy, George Washington University School of Medicine and Health Sciences, Washington, D.C. 20037; Veterans Administration Medical Center, Washington, D.C. 20422

Truvor Kuzmowych, M.D., Assistant Professor of Medicine, Division of Pulmonary Diseases and Allergy, George Washington University School of Medicine and Health Sciences, Washington, D.C. 20037; Chief, Pulmonary Clinic, Veterans Administration Medical Center, Washington, D.C. 20422

Ann Medinger, M.D., F.A.C.P., F.C.C.P., Assistant Professor of Medicine, Division of Pulmonary Diseases and Allergy, George Washington University School of Medicine and Health Sciences, Washington, D.C. 20037; Chief, Pulmonary Function Laboratory, Veterans Administration Medical Center, Washington, D.C. 20422

Prashant Rohatgi, M.D., Associate Chief, Pulmonary Disease Section, Veterans Administration Medical Center, Washington, D.C. 20422; Associate Professor of Medicine, Division of Pulmonary Diseases and Allergy, George Washington University School of Medicine and Health Sciences, Washington, D.C. 20037

Sorell L. Schwartz, Ph.D., Professor of Pharmacology, Georgetown University Schools of Medicine and Dentistry, Washington, D.C. 20007;

Scientific Director, Center for Environmental Health and Human Toxicology, Washington, D.C. 20007

Samuel V. Spagnolo, M.D., F.A.C.P., F.C.C.P., Professor of Medicine, Director, Division of Pulmonary Diseases and Allergy, Associate Chairman, Department of Medicine, George Washington University School of Medicine and Health Sciences, Washington, D.C. 20037; Chief, Pulmonary Disease Section, Veterans Administration Medical Center, Washington, D.C. 20422

Philip Witorsch, M.D., F.A.C.P., F.C.C.P., Clinical Professor of Medicine, Associate Director, Respiratory Care, Division of Pulmonary Diseases and Allergy, George Washington University School of Medicine and Health Sciences, Washington, D.C. 20037; Adjunct Professor of Pharmacology, Georgetown University Schools of Medicine and Dentistry, Washington, D.C. 20007; Medical Director, Center for Environmental Health and Human Toxicology, Washington, D.C. 20007

Preface

This book is written for medical students and house officers working on the wards, in the intensive care unit, and in the emergency room. It is intended for use by all whose work involves the daily evaluation and management of medical emergencies.

The material is a compilation of information gained from our personal experiences in clinical practice, from participation in professional meetings and conferences, and from searching the medical literature.

The introductory chapters in Part I form a foundation that is developed in the subsequent parts where specific topics are discussed. When possible, we have simplified complex approaches to diagnosis and management by formulating algorithms and handy reference tables.

Since this is a handbook and not a textbook, we have limited our discussion of pathogenesis and pathophysiology in order to concentrate on practical aspects and specific details that are useful in the diagnosis and management of pulmonary emergencies. Our aim is to alert young physicians to common pulmonary emergencies and guide them through their initial management.

ACKNOWLEDGMENTS. We owe much to our contributors, colleagues, and students, who gave us ideas for this book over many years. Our thanks to the husbands, wives, and friends of the contributors; they have given of their time so that these chapters could be completed. Finally, our special thanks to Ms. Anita Seidl, Ms. Sherri Long, Ms. Beverly Parsons, and Ms. Maria Melendez for assisting in the preparation of the chapters, and to Ms. Margaret Evans for typing and organizing the final manuscript.

Samuel V. Spagnolo
Ann Medinger

Washington, D.C.

Contents

Part I. The Approach to Patient Evaluation

Chapter 1
Clinical Assessment of the Patient with Pulmonary Disease
Samuel V. Spagnolo

Chapter 2
Interpretation of Arterial Blood Gases in the Emergency Patient
Ann Medinger

Part II. Normal Lungs with Acute Respiratory Decompensation

Chapter 3
Extrapulmonic Ventilatory Failure
Ann Medinger

Chapter 4
Life-Threatening Pneumonia
Morgan D. Delaney, Samuel V. Spagnolo, and Ann Medinger

Chapter 5
Acute Inhalation Lung Disease
Philip Witorsch and Sorell L. Schwartz

Chapter 6
Pulmonary Edema
Philip Witorsch and Ann Medinger

Chapter 7
Near-Drowning
Kenneth Dickie

Chapter 8
Chest Trauma
Truvor Kuzmowych

Chapter 9
Upper-Airway Emergencies
Kenneth Dickie

Part III. Chronic Lung Disease with Acute Respiratory
Decompensation

Chapter 10
Acute Respiratory Failure in the Patient
with Chronic Airflow Obstruction
Samuel V. Spagnolo

Chapter 11
Asthma
Morgan D. Delaney

Part IV. Pulmonary Vascular Emergencies

Chapter 12
Hemoptysis
Truvor Kuzmowych and Samuel V. Spagnolo

Chapter 13
Embolic Pulmonary Disease
Aram A. Arabian

Chapter 14
Superior Vena Cava Syndrome
Prashant Rohatgi

Part V. Pleural Emergencies

Chapter 15
Catastrophic Pleural Disease
Prashant Rohagti

Part VI. Ventilator Emergencies

Chapter 16
Ventilatory Assistance and Its Complications
Aram A. Arabian, Ann Medinger, and Samuel V. Spagnolo

Appendix A
Terms and Symbols

Appendix B
Normal Values

Handbook of
Pulmonary
Emergencies

The Approach to Patient Evaluation

CLINICAL SIGNS AND SYMPTOMS OF PULMONARY DISEASE

Patients with pulmonary disease may develop one or more of the following signs or symptoms:

- Cough
- Sputum production
- Chest pain
- Dyspnea
- Wheezing
- Cyanosis
- Hemoptysis

Cough

Great care should be taken to elicit a history of cough. Many patients do not readily admit to coughing or may be unaware of its importance. Coughing is considered a part of a ''normal'' daily life by some individuals. Worsening of a chronic cough may be a clue to the development of new disease. The most common causes of cough are

- Smoking
- Asthma
- Respiratory infection
- Lung cancer

The type of cough should be noted:

Examples of Coughs

Type	Possible cause(s)
Dry, irritative	Toxic gas injury, lung cancer
Productive	Acute lung infection
Morning only	Smoking, sinusitis
Nocturnal only	Asthma, heart disease
Positional	Esophageal disorders, lung abscess

Sputum Production

Normal persons produce less than 100 ml of lower-respiratory-tract secretions daily. Production of larger amounts indicates disease and frequently leads to expectoration. Sputum production should be carefully characterized as to

- Onset
- Amount
- Color

- Frequency
- Precipitating and relieving factors (such as the patient's position)

Examples of Sputum Production

Type	Possible cause(s)
Thick, white, daily sputum	Chronic bronchitis
Yellow and/or blood tinged	Acute respiratory infection, lung cancer
Black pigment visible	Anthracosis

Chest Pain

No symptom produces more anxiety in patients than chest pain, but the causes are many. Chest pain should be characterized as follows:

- Acute or gradual onset
- Sharp or dull
- Occurs or worsens with deep breathing (pleuritic)
- Localized or diffuse
- Precipitating factors
- Relieving factors
- Associated signs and symptoms
- Radiation
- Duration of each episode

Chest pain evaluated in the above manner will help in determining the exact cause:

Examples of Chest Pain

Type	Possible cause(s)
Gradual onset, dull pain	Lung cancer, lung abscess
Acute onset, sharp, localized pain	Lung infection
Acute onset, pleuritic pain	Pulmonary embolus, lung infection

Dyspnea

Breathing perceived by the patient to be difficult, uncomfortable, or unpleasant is defined as dyspnea.

The reasons for dyspnea are complex and some are speculative. Dyspnea usually results from abnormal lung mechanics (e.g., lungs that are stiff from increased interstitial water or tissue or that have airflow obstruction). Mediastinal abnormalities may also produce dyspnea. Dyspnea at rest indicates severe disease. Dyspnea with exertion or exercise suggests less severe disease. Dyspnea should be characterized as follows:

- Onset
- Positional
- Nocturnal
- Effort related
- Frequency
- Precipitating factors
- Relieving factors

Examples of Dyspnea

Type	Possible cause(s)
Acute dyspnea with wheezing	Acute asthhma, pulmonary embolus
Acute dyspnea with chest pain, fever, and productive cough	Acute pneumonia
Gradual onset of dyspnea without cough	Interstitial lung fibrosis
Dyspnea relieved by sitting position	Left heart disease

Wheezing

Wheezing indicates airway obstruction and has many causes. It can result from primary pulmonary disease or from cardiac disease with secondary lung involvement. A wheeze on inspiration is often referred to as *stridor* and commonly signifies extrathoracic airway obstruction. Remember "all that wheezes is not asthma."

Evaluate wheezing as follows:

- Unilateral
- Bilateral
- Constant
- Onset (abrupt or gradual)
- Associated finding (e.g., fever, chest pain, sputum production)

Examples of Wheezing

Type	Possible cause(s)
Unilateral wheeze	Bronchial adenoma, foreign body
Acute, bilateral	Pulmonary embolus, asthma

Hemoptysis

Hemoptysis is always important and requires evaluation; never treat it casually. Although in many patients the exact etiology of the bleeding will not be determined, each recurrent episode requires complete evaluation because new treatable bleeding sources appear in previous bleeders, and lesions that may go undetected with the first bleed often become evident later. An effort should be made to identify the source of the blood, distinguishing particularly the upper airway, the esophagus, and the lower respiratory tract (LRT) as sources. LRT hemoptysis tends to recur at least once or twice. Occasionally, patients will be able to localize the site of bleeding to one side of the chest themselves. Acute life-threatening hemoptysis is reviewed in Chapter 12.

Cyanosis

Cyanosis may be present with mild to moderate hypoxemia; when present, it demands ABG confirmation of the state of blood oxygenation. In the presence of severe anemia, cyanosis may be absent even with severe hypoxemia. Cyanosis may be associated with

- Severe hypoxemia
- Methemoglobinemia
- Sulfhemoglobinemia

ADDITIONAL CLINICAL INFORMATION

Other Symptoms

It is important to search for additional symptoms, signs, and historical information. These include

- Fever [oral temperature greater than 100.4°F (38°C)]
- Chills
- Diaphoresis
- Weight loss
- Hoarseness
- Joint or bone pain
- Dysphagia
- Clubbing of fingers and toes

Although the above are frequently nonspecific items, when present in association with the symptoms already discussed, they greatly assist in making the specific pulmonary diagnosis.

Examples of Other Signs and Symptoms

Type	Possible cause(s)
Cough, fever, chest x ray infiltrates, and dysphagia	Esophageal disease: for example • Cancer • Stricture • Diverticula • Motility disorder
Cough, hemoptysis, and joint pain	Lung cancer
Fever, cough, mass on chest x ray, and clubbing	Lung cancer with postobstructive pneumonia, lung abscess
Fever, hoarseness, cavitary infiltrate on chest x-ray	Pulmonary and laryngeal tuberculosis

TABLE 1. Drugs Reported to Produce Lung Abnormalities

Aminorex	Melphalan
Aminosalicylate	Mephenesin
Amiodarone	Methadone
Amitriptyline	Methotrexate
Aspirin (acetylsalicylic acid)	Methyldopa
Azathioprine	Methysergide maleate
	Mitomycin-C
Bleomycin	
Busulfan	Naproxen
	Nitrofurantoin
Carmustine (BCNU)	
Chlorambucil	Paraldehyde
Chlorpropamide	Penicillamine
Cromolyn sodium	Penicillin
Cytosine arabinoside (Ara-C)	Phenylbutazone
	Phenytoin
Ethchlorvynol	Pindolol
	Procainamide
Fenoprofen	Procarbazine hydrochloride
	Propoxyphene hydrochloride
Gold	Propranolol
Griseofulvin	
	Salicylate
Hexamethonium	Semustine (methyl-CCNU)
Hydrochlorothiazide	Sulindac
	Sulphasalazine
Ibuprofen	
Imipramine hydrochloride	Tetracycline
Indomethacin	Tolmetin
Iodine preparations	
Isoniazid	Uracil mustard
Marijuana	Zinostatin
Mercaptopurine	Zomepirac

Drug and/or Medication Use

Over-the-counter, physician prescribed, or illicit drug ingestion, injection, or inhalation may lead to acute or chronic pulmonary disease. The list of offending agents is long and includes examples from almost all classes of drugs. Pulmonary reactions to these agents range from acute hypersensitivity to direct "toxic" injury to the alveolar–capillary membrane. A listing of these agents can be found in Table 1.

Toxic Chemical Exposure

The subject of toxic chemical injury to the lung is discussed in Chapter 5.

PHYSICAL EXAMINATION

Initial Appearance

The physical examination begins when you first observe the patient by noting

- General appearance
- Mental state (alert, somnolent, coma)
- Signs of fever, diaphoresis
- Breathing pattern (depth, frequency, type)
- Signs of respiratory distress
    - Use of accessory muscles
    - Flaring of alae nasi on inspiration
    - Noisy breathing or wheezing
    - Cough and sputum production

This initial visual part of the examination can take place rapidly and without even touching the patient.

Vital Signs

Vital signs should be obtained and the physical examination should focus on the following organ systems:

- Lymph nodes: for enlargement (especially supraclavicular, cervical, and axillary)

- Fingers and toes: for clubbing, cyanosis
- Eyes: for extraocular evidence of Horner's syndrome (metastatic malignancy) and for retinal evidence of choroidal tubercles (clue to the diagnosis of miliary tuberculosis)
- Neck vessels: for evaluation of venous pressure (right-heart failure; superior vena cava syndrome)
- Chest wall and lungs: this part of the examination should be done over all thoracic areas, anteriorly and posteriorly
  - Inspection for signs to previous surgery, trauma, or deformity
  - Palpation to determine resonance or dullness
  - Percussion to determine resonance or dullness
  - Auscultation to determine presence of:
    - Wheezing
    - Ronchi
    - Crackles (early, late, fine, or harsh)
    - Decreased, increased, or absent breath sounds
- Diaphragm: measurement of movement bilaterally at full inspiration and expiration
- Pleura: friction rubs may be located in very small circumscribed areas and, unless searched for, are easily missed
- Heart: the examination of the pulmonary system is not complete without thorough inspection, palpation, percussion, and auscultation of the heart, where findings may be found that will help determine whether the pulmonary disease is related to either right and/or left-heart abnormalities

LABORATORY ASSESSMENT

Chest X Ray

In evaluating a patient with possible pulmonary disease, a chest x ray must be obtained in all cases. The chest x ray should include both a standard posterior–anterior and a lateral chest x ray (when a patient is seen for the first time). Many abnormalities that are not apparent from history or physical examination are revealed by the chest x ray. Occasionally, the chest roentgenogram itself has such distinctive diagnostic features that the diagnosis seems certain.

For example:

- Diffuse radiodense pattern of occupational lung disease such as
  - Baritosis

- ○ Silicosis
- ○ Stannosis
- • Well-defined, multiple "cannonball" *masses* from metastatic tumor such as
  - ○ Testicular
  - ○ Renal
- • Discrete, widespread nodular calcifications from
  - ○ Chicken pox
  - ○ Histoplasmosis
- • Bilateral, symmetrical hilar nodes with right paratracheal node enlargement from
  - ○ Sarcoidosis
- • Frequently, lung infections may give characteristic but not necessarily unique appearance, such as cavitary infiltrates
  - ○ Tuberculosis
  - ○ Coccidioidomycosis
  - ○ Histoplasmosis

Many exceptions to the above can be found, and in *no* instance should a final diagnosis be made without additional confirmatory information. In the case of pneumoconiosis, the additional confirmatory evidence may simply be a relevant history of occupational exposure.

Sputum Examination

If the patient is producing sputum, appropriate stains, such as Gram and acid-fast, should be performed on a fresh specimen and the slides examined for bacteria and mycobacteria. The unstained sputum (wet mount preparation) should also be examined microscopically for

- • Polymorphonuclear white blood cells (infection)
- • Eosinophils (hypersensitivity)
- • Charcot-Leyden crystals (asthma)
- • Curschmann's spirals (asthma)

The gram stain has great importance in identifying the organism in cases of respiratory infection because of

- • Speed
- • Upper airway bacterial contamination of sputum cultures may lead to difficulty in interpreting culture results

Samples of sputum should also be sent fresh to the laboratory for selective cultures and cytology. When sputum is not obtainable or is unreliable and infection is suspected, material may be obtained from the lower respiratory tract by percutaneous lung aspiration or by translaryngeal aspiration; it should be cultured for both aerobic and anaerobic bacteria. (See Chapter 4, Life-Threatening Pneumonia).

ABG

ABG should be measured in all patients with pulmonary or cardiovascular emergencies, and in all pulmonary patients with a history of previous lung infection, such as tuberculosis, recurring pneumonia, or previous lung surgery. It is clinically impossible to determine when mild-to-moderate hypoxemia exists. Cyanosis may be apparent only when there are severe degrees of hypoxemia. Other laboratory findings that may suggest the presence of underlying chronic hypoxemia and the need for ABG include

- Elevated hematocrit
- Elevated hemoglobin
- Elevated serum bicarbonate
- Low serum chloride
- Electrocardiogram showing right-heart strain or right-axis deviation

Pulmonary Function Tests

Tests available include

- Spirometry and flow-volume loops
- Lung volumes
- Lung compliance
- Airway resistance

For measuring airflow obstruction, the best tests are

- FEV_1
- FVC
- Flow-volume loops

For patients with restrictive pulmonary abnormalities, the best tests are

- Vital capacity
- Total lung capacity

- Diffusing capacity for carbon monoxide $D_L CO$
- Exercise ABG

In patients with severe but *stable* lung disease, little benefit is gained from frequent pulmonary function testing.

Tests are now available to investigate central nervous system abnormalities in control of ventilation.

Special Laboratory Studies

Other special studies available for the evaluation of these acutely ill pulmonary patients include

- Fiberoptic bronchoscopy with
  - Transbronchial lung biopsy
  - Wang needle biopsy of subcarinal nodes
  - Bronchial brushing
  - Bronchial biopsy
  - Broncho–alveolar lavage
- Thoracentesis fluid for
  - Chemistry
  - Cytology
  - Culture for microorganisms
- Pleural biopsy for
  - Histology
  - Culture for microorganisms
- Percutaneous lung aspiration for
  - Cytology
  - Culture of microorganisms
- Open lung biopsy via thoracotomy for
  - Histology
  - Culture of microorganisms
- Pleuroscopy (thoracoscopy)
- Translaryngeal aspiration
- Skin testing

These special studies are required when other less invasive methods have failed to yield a diagnosis. The results of these tests used in conjunction with information obtained from other sources will enable the clinician to make a diagnosis, assess the degree of functional impairment, and guide management.

INDICATIONS FOR HOSPITALIZATION OF THE PATIENT WITH PULMONARY DISEASE

Guidelines that I have found useful in determining the need for hospitalization are listed below. Most items will require extensive, prompt evaluation and treatment.

- Confusion, severe anxiety, or personality change
- Labored breathing
- Chest pain with hemoptysis
- Cyanosis
- Intractable bronchospasm
- Inability to raise pulmonary secretions
- Smoke inhalation with elevated carboxyhemoglobin levels
- Severely disturbed sleep owing to cough, wheezing, or dyspnea
- Toxic patient with pneumonia
- Hemoptysis of 100 ml or more
- Suspected pulmonary embolus
- Penetrating chest injury
- Crushing chest injury
- New pleural effusion
- ABG values:
  - Pa_{O_2} less than 50 mm Hg
  - Pa_{CO_2} greater than 55 mm Hg
  - pH less than 7.30

INDICATIONS FOR HOSPITALIZATION OF THE PATIENT WITH PULMONARY DISEASE

CHAPTER 2

Interpretation of Arterial Blood Gases in the Emergency Patient

Ann Medinger

Arterial blood gas (ABG) analysis is a critical element in the modern diagnosis and management of pulmonary emergencies. There are no clinical · findings that correlate specifically and well with pH, Pa_{CO_2}, and Pa_{O_2} measurements. Knowledge of the abnormalities in pH, Pa_{O_2}, and Pa_{CO_2} allows the physician to direct early therapeutic and diagnostic efforts with the greatest lifesaving efficiency. Normal values are given in Appendix B.

SOURCE OF BLOOD FOR ABG ANALYSIS

The blood sample for gas analysis may be taken from a systemic artery, the main pulmonary artery, or a cardiac chamber. Gas analysis from each of these sites gives different information. The *systemic artery* ABG reflects overall pulmonary function; the *main pulmonary artery* ABG tells how well the tissues are extracting oxygen; the *intracardiac* ABG tells whether intracardiac anatomic shunts are present. For the purposes of this chapter, arterial blood gas (ABG) analysis will refer to samples from a systemic artery.

Ann Medinger • Division of Pulmonary Diseases and Allergy, George Washington University School of Medicine and Health Sciences, Washington, D.C. 20037; Pulmonary Function Laboratory, Veterans Administration Medical Center, Washington, D.C. 20422.

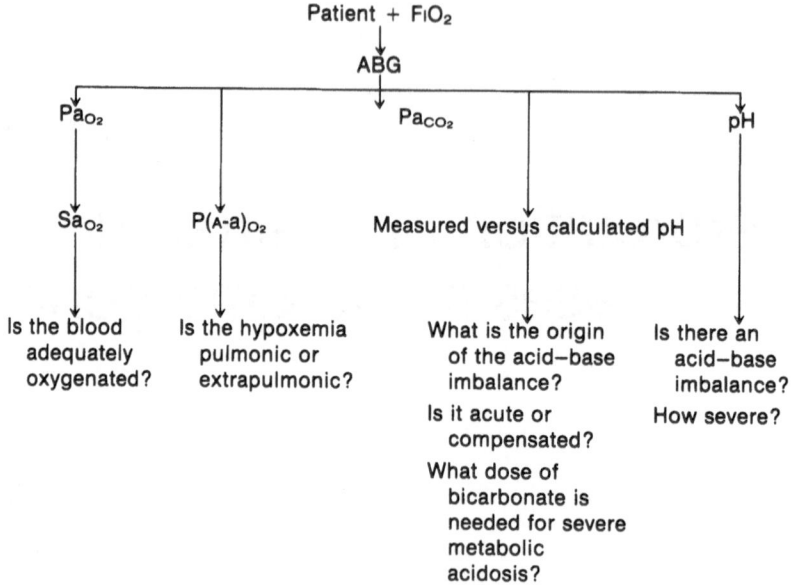

FIGURE 1. Algorithm for analyzing the ABG.

USES OF ABG MEASUREMENTS

Blood gas measurements give early and continuing information about four important aspects of the body's life support system:

- The state of *oxygenation*
- The presence of *injury to the lung*
- The *acid–base balance*
- The *cause of hydrogen excess or deficit*, whether predominantly a respiratory or metabolic malfunction

The use of the ABG to define these aspects is summarized in Fig. 1. The following sections outline the simple manipulations of pH, Pa_{O_2}, and Pa_{CO_2} values that are needed to get the most information from the ABG.

OXYGENATION AND THE ABG

The Pa_{O_2} tells whether the patient's *blood* is being adequately oxygenated by his lungs. The Pa_{O_2} alone does not tell whether the patient's *tissues*—heart, brain, and kidney—are getting enough oxygen.

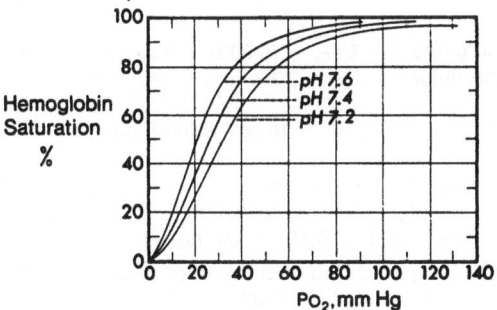

FIGURE 2. Oxyhemoglobin dissociation curve.

Blood Oxygenation

The Pa_{O_2} is an indirect indicator of adequate *blood oxygenation* (Ca_{O_2}) The Pa_{O_2} tells how much oxygen is dissolved in the blood. However, only 1–2% of the blood's total oxygen content is in the dissolved form. Ninety-eight percent of the blood's oxygen is carried by hemoglobin (Hb). The degree to which the Hb is saturated with oxygen (Sa_{O_2}) and hence the blood oxygen content (Ca_{O_2}), can be estimated from the Pa_{O_2} by referring to the normal oxyhemoglobin dissociation curve (see Fig. 2), and assuming the Hb concentration is normal, 15 ($Ca_{O_2} \cong 1.38 \times$ Hb $\times$ Sa_{O_2}; 1.38 is the oxyhemoglobin combining coefficient).

In the emergency patient, the blood may be considered adequately oxygenated by the lungs if the Pa_{O_2} is high enough to saturate the Hb 90% with oxygen ($Sa_{O_2} = 90\%$). Normally, this occurs when the Pa_{O_2} is 60 mm Hg. (see Fig. 2). However, if there is acidosis and/or fever (which shifts the oxyhemoglobin curve to the right), a Pa_{O_2} of 70 mm Hg may be required to adequately oxygenate the blood ($Sa_{O_2} \geq 90\%$).

Tissue Oxygenation

Adequate oxygenation of the patient's blood does not assure adequate oxygenation of the patient's heart, brain, and kidneys. *Tissue oxygenation* depends on the transport of the oxygenated blood and the extraction of the oxygen by the tissues. Figure 3 outlines the factors that determine oxygen transport to and extraction by the tissues.

A Pa_{O_2} measurement greater than 60 mm Hg, probably confirms adequate blood oxygenation, as well as adequate oxygenation of the patient's tissues if

- Pulse and blood pressure are normal or increased (adequate cardiac output)

Equations

Blood oxygen content = Ca_{O_2} = $(0.0031 \times Pa_{O_2}) + (1.38 \times Sa_{O_2} \times Hb)$

Tissue oxygen uptake = $\dot{V}_{O_2}$ = $13.8 \times \dot{Q} \times Hb \times (Sa_{O_2} - S\bar{v}_{O_2})$

$\qquad\qquad\qquad\qquad$ (heart) (blood) (lungs) (tissue extraction)

Example

Pa_{O_2} = 60 mm Hg; Sa_{O_2} = 0.90; $S\bar{v}_{O_2}$ = 0.45; $\dot{Q}$ = 4 liters/min; Hb = 10

Ca_{O_2} = $(0.0031 \times 60) + (1.38 \times 0.9 \times 10)$ = 0.186 + 12.42 = 12.6 mm

$\dot{V}_{O_2}$ = $13.8 \times 4 \times 10 (0.9 - 0.45)$ = 248 ml/min

Assessment: 1. Oxygen content is reduced (normal = 20), primarily due to reduced Hb (normal = 15).

2. Although $\dot{Q}$ is also reduced (normal = 5), $\dot{V}_{O_2}$ is normal because of a compensatory increase in tissue oxygen extraction (normal $S\bar{v}_{O_2}$ = 0.75).

Plan: Direct therapy toward improving Hb and $\dot{Q}$.

FIGURE 3. Factors determining tissue oxygenation. $S\bar{v}$ = oxygen saturation of hemoglobin in mixed venous blood; Sa_{O_2} = oxygen saturation of hemoglobin in arterial blood; Hb = hemoglobin concentration; $\dot{Q}$ = cardiac output; 0.0031 = solubility coefficient for oxygen in blood; 1.38 = oxyhemoglobin-combining coefficient; 13.8 = oxyhemoglobin-combining coefficient $\times$ unit conversion factor.

- No pallor of mucous membranes (adequate Hb)
- No fever or acidosis (normal O_2–Hb curve)
- Mentally alert or good urine output (adequate O_2 extraction)

LUNG INJURY AND THE ABG

Hypoxemia is a reduced Pa_{O_2} (below 80 mm Hg at sea level). When hypoxemia is present, calculation of the $P(A\text{-}a)_{O_2}$ from the ABG (described below) is the simplest means of identifying or confirming lung injury as the cause of the low Pa_{O_2}.

Hypoxemia, Differential Diagnosis

The five physiologic derangements that cause *hypoxemia* are

- *Ventilation–perfusion imbalance*—mismatching of the blood and airflow to the lung
- *Right-to-left shunt*—wasted blood, flowing to the left heart (systemic circulation) without receiving oxygen
- *Diffusion impairment*—thickening of the alveolar–capillary interface between blood and air

TABLE 1. The Differential Diagnosis of Hypoxemia[a]

Pulmonic	1. Ventilation–perfusion imbalance
	    Asthma, CAO, pulmonary embolism
	2. Right-to-left blood shunt
	    Pneumonia, ARDS, cardiac or vascular malformations
	3. Diffusion impairment
	    Interstitial fibrosis, lymphatic obstruction

Extrapulmonic	4. Hypoventilation
	    Sedative overdose, organophosphate poisoning, amyotrophic
	    lateral sclerosis
	5. Low PI_{O_2}
	    High altitude, erroneus gas mixtures given during controlled or
	    assisted ventilation

[a] CAO = chronic airflow obstruction; ARDS = adult respiratory distress syndrome; PI_{O_2} = partial pressure of inspired oxygen.

- *Hypoventilation*—inadequate air delivery to and from perfused alveoli
- *Low PI_{O_2}*—inadequate partial pressure of inspired oxygen caused by breathing an hypoxic gas mixture or by breathing air with low total barometric pressure.

Table 1 lists examples of hypoxic diseases according to the primary cause of the hypoxemia. Frequently, more than one physiologic derangement is present; for example, patients with chronic airway obstruction may have predominant ventilation–perfusion imbalance, which is accompanied by hypoventilation. Diffusion impairment causes such mild reductions in the Pa_{O_2} that it will not be further considered in this section. Each of these physiologic derangements calls for different treatment to correct the hypoxemia. Appropriate specific treatment is discussed in subsequent chapters.

$P(A\text{-}a)_{O_2}$ Differentiation of Hypoxemic Diseases

The $P(A\text{-}a)_{O_2}$, which is simply calculated from the ABG values, distinguishes *pulmonic* (groups 1 and 2, Table 1) from *extrapulmonic* (groups 3 and 4, Table 1) causes of hypoxemia. The $P(A\text{-}a)_{O_2}$ is elevated in pulmonic and normal in extrapulmonic derangements causing hypoxemia.

The $P(A\text{-}a)_{O_2}$ is a measure of the difference between the PA_{O_2} in the alveolar space and the Pa_{O_2} in the arterial space. Any derangement of the lung that disrupts either blood flow or airflow will raise the $P(A\text{-}a)_{O_2}$. The arterial Pa_{O_2} is measured in the arterial blood sample. Since it is not possible to sample alveolar air, the alveolar PA_{O_2} is calculated from the alveolar air equation. The $P(A\text{-}a)_{O_2}$ can be estimated by means

Equation: $P(\text{A-a})_{O_2} = (\text{B.P.} - 47) \times F_{I_{O_2}} - \dfrac{Pa_{CO_2}}{0.8} - Pa_{O_2}$

Sea level simplification: $P(\text{A-a})_{O_2} \cong 700 \times F_{I_{O_2}} - \left(\dfrac{Pa_{CO_2}}{0.8}\right) - Pa_{O_2}$

Examples:

1. $Pa_{O_2} = 65$ mm Hg; $Pa_{CO_2} = 60$ mm Hg; pH = 7.24
   $F_{I_{O_2}} = 0.21$ (room air); B.P. = 750 (sea level)

   $P(\text{A-a})_{O_2} = (750 - 47) \times 0.21 - \left(\dfrac{60}{0.8}\right) - 65$

   $\cong 700 \times 0.21 - 75 - 65$

   $\cong 7$

   Assessment: $P(\text{A-a})_{O_2}$ is normal (<25); therefore, hypoxemia (normal Pa_{O_2} 80–100) is due to an extrapulmonic problem. The elevated Pa_{CO_2} confirms that hypoventilation is causing the problem. Extrapulmonic ventilatory failure (see Chapter 3) is the diagnosis.

2. $Pa_{O_2} = 60$ mm Hg; $Pa_{CO_2} = 30$ mm Hg; pH = 7.48
   $F_{I_{O_2}} = 0.4$ (breathing 40% Venturi mask); B.P. = 760 (sea level)

   $P(\text{A-a})_{O_2} = (760 - 47) \times 0.4 - \left(\dfrac{30}{0.8}\right) - 60$

   $\cong (700 \times 0.4) - 37 - 60$

   $\cong 182.5$

   Assessment: $P(\text{A-a})_{O_2}$ is increased; hypoxemia is due to either ventilation–perfusion mismatch or a right-to-left shunt. Repeating the ABG with patient breathing 100% O_2 would distinguish these two.

FIGURE 4. Calculation of the alveolar–arterial oxygen gradient, $P(\text{A-a})_{O_2}$. $F_{I_{O_2}}$ = fraction of inhaled O_2; B.P. = barometric pressure. See text for explanation of equations.

of the following equation:

$$P(\text{A-a})_{O_2} = (\text{B.P.} - 47) \times F_{I_{O_2}} - \frac{Pa_{CO_2}}{0.8} - Pa_{O_2}$$

(In this equation B.P. is barometric pressure in mm Hg; 47 is the tracheal water vapor pressure in mm Hg; $F_{I_{O_2}}$ is the fraction of inspired oxygen; and 0.8 is the normal respiratory exchange quotient.) Two physiologic assumptions are implicit in this computation: first, that the alveolar and arterial P_{CO_2} are equal, and second, that the ratio of exchange of carbon dioxide and oxygen ($\dot{v}_{CO_2}/\dot{v}_{O_2}$) across the lung is normal, 0.8. See Fig. 4 for examples illustrating the computation and use of the $P(\text{A-a})_{O_2}$.

A summary of the use of the ABG to find the cause of hypoxemia and implications of this analysis for therapy are given in the algorithm of Fig. 5.

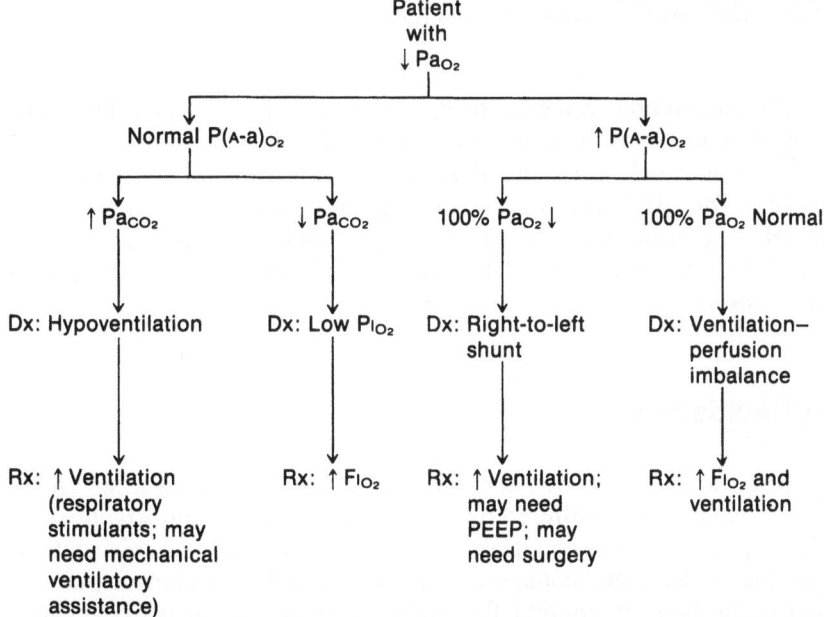

FIGURE 5. Using the ABG to evaluate and treat hypoxemia: role of the $P(A-a)_{O_2}$. $P(A-a)_{O_2}$ = alveolar–arterial oxygen difference = (B.P. − 47) × $F_{I_{O_2}}$ − ($Pa_{CO_2}/0.8$) − Pa_{O_2}; Dx = diagnosis; Rx = therapy; $P_{I_{O_2}}$ = partial pressure of inspired oxygen; $F_{I_{O_2}}$ = fraction of inspired oxygen; PEEP = positive end-expiratory pressure.

Hypoxemia due to Pulmonic Diseases

An *increased* $P(A-a)_{O_2}$ (>25 mm Hg) in hypoxemic patients indicates the presence of *pulmonic impairment*. The ABG also permits differentiation of patients with significant right-to-left shunts from the rest with ventilation–perfusion impairment. When the ABG is repeated with the patient breathing 100% oxygen, patients with a significant right-to-left shunt are found to have a lower-than-expected Pa_{O_2} (<500 mm Hg).

Hypoxemia due to Extrapulmonic Diseases

A *normal* $P(A-a)_{O_2}$ (<25 mm Hg) in hypoxemic patients indicates the presence of *extrapulmonic impairment*. Those who are hypoventilating may be distinguished from those with a reduced $P_{I_{O_2}}$ by an elevated Pa_{CO_2}.

ACID–BASE BALANCE AND THE ABG

The human body's metabolic processes require a pH of 7.40 ± 0.04 for optimal function. Cellular life is impaired by alterations in this normal pH, and values below 6.8 and above 7.8 are not compatible with continuing life. The pH is a representation of the concentration of hydrogen ions [H+]; it is the negative log of [H+]. Hence, a rise in pH reflects a fall in [H+], and vice versa. The normal pH 7.40 reflects an [H+] of 40 nanamoles/liter.

Sources of Acidemia

Acidemia occurs when the pH falls below 7.36; it signifies an increased number of unbuffered hydrogen ions in circulation. *Alkalemia* is a rise in pH over 7.44 and signifies reduced hydrogen ions in circulation. Acidemia is the more common acid–base disorder in clinical practice because the body is continually producing metabolic acid by-products which must be eliminated. The rate of production of these acids may increase, as occurs in strenuous exercise (lactate) and uncontrolled diabetes mellitus (β-hydroxybuterate). The lungs and the kidneys are the principal excretors of metabolic acid by-products. This excretion of metabolic acids may be impaired by failure of either of these excretory organs. Hence, acidemia develops from overproduction or underexcretion. It may also arise from pathologic ingestion of exogenous acids, such as methanol (canned heat) or ethylene glycol (antifreeze).

Renal and Respiratory Compensation for Acid–Base Imbalance

Normally, mild impairment of acid excretion by either the lungs or kidneys is compensated by increased acid removal by the other organ.

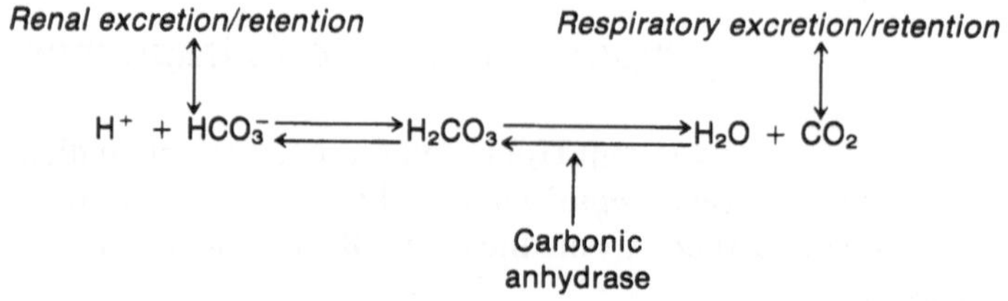

Renal excretion/retention   Respiratory excretion/retention

$$H^+ + HCO_3^- \rightleftharpoons H_2CO_3 \rightleftharpoons H_2O + CO_2$$

Carbonic
anhydrase

FIGURE 6. Bicarbonate—the labile body buffer.

This compensated impairment may be detected in the ABG measurement even when the pH remains normal. It is called *acidosis* (tendency toward low pH) or *alkalosis* (tendency toward high pH); it may be respiratory or metabolic, depending on the origin of imbalance.

FINDING THE ORIGIN OF ACID–BASE IMBALANCE WITH THE ABG

Renal and respiratory systems not only eliminate most metabolic acid by-products, but also control the principal labile blood buffer, *the bicarbonate buffer system* (see Fig. 6).

The relationship between the blood's pH and the elements of this bicarbonate buffering system is expressed by the Henderson–Hasselbach equation (see Fig. 7). The Pa_{CO_2} is the respiratory component; the $[HCO_3^-]$ is the renal metabolic component. As long as the ratio of $[HCO_3^-]/(0.03 \times Pa_{CO_2})$ remains 20/1, pH will be normal, i.e., 7.40. Note that the absolute values of $[HCO_3^-]$ and Pa_{CO_2} are far less important in regulating pH than the ratio of the two. Note also that changing the Pa_{CO_2} has an opposite effect on pH; changing the $[HCO_3^-]$ has a direct effect on pH. Using this information to assess the emergency patient will often identify the origin and the components of the acid–base disorder.

$$\text{Equation: pH} = 6.1 + \log \frac{[HCO_3^-]}{[H_2CO_3]} = 6.1 + \log \frac{[HCO_3^-]}{0.03 \times Pa_{CO_2}}$$

$$\text{pH} = 6.1 + \log \frac{20}{1} = 6.1 + 1.3 = 7.4$$

Conclusions:

1. $\text{pH} \propto \dfrac{\text{renal control of } [HCO_3^-]}{\text{respiratory control of } Pa_{CO_2}}$

2. Since $Pa_{CO_2} \propto \dfrac{1}{\text{ventilation}}$, and

   $[HCO_3^-] \propto$ renal excretion:

3. pH $\propto$ minute ventilation and

   pH $\propto$ renal bicarbonate excretion

FIGURE 7. Modified Henderson–Hasselbach equation: renal and respiratory relationship. 6.1 = dissociation constant for the bicarbonate buffering system; 0.03 = constant term relating $[H_2CO_3]$ and Pa_{CO_2}; 20/1 = normal plasma ratio of $[HCO_3^-]/0.03 \times Pa_{CO_2}$; 7.4 = normal blood pH.

Identifying the Respiratory Component of Acid–Base Imbalance

The pH and Pa_{CO_2} alone tell whether there is a *respiratory contribution* to the acid–base problem:

- pH deviation from normal opposite from Pa_{CO_2} deviation—respiratory impairment
- pH deviation from normal same as Pa_{CO_2} deviation—no respiratory impairment

The pH and Pa_{CO_2} also tell about the *severity of the disorder*:

- pH less than 7.20 and greater than 7.65 signifies severe acid–base imbalance
- Pa_{CO_2} greater than 55 mm Hg signifies severe respiratory impairment

Assessment of the relationship of pH to Pa_{CO_2} is not sufficient to detect the presence or predominance of a metabolic component. To do this you must compute the calculated pH and compare it to the measured pH.

The Calculated pH for Source Identification

Using the Henderson–Hasselbach equation to compute the pH deviation that is attributable to the measured Pa_{CO_2} gives the *calculated pH* and allows identification of

- Probable *origin* of the acid–base imbalance
- *Respiratory and metabolic* components of mixed disorders
- The *degree of compensation* by the nonimpaired organ

The calculated pH (pH_c) is computed with the following simple Hendersin–Hasselbach-derived formula:

$$pH_c = 7.40 - 0.008 \times [Pa_{CO_2} - 40]$$

(In this formula 7.40 is the normal blood pH; 40 is the normal blood Pa_{CO_2} in mm Hg; and 0.008 is the expected change in pH for each 1-mm change in Pa_{CO_2}, at a constant bicarbonate concentration.) Since the variance of calculated from measured pH is due to $[HCO_3^-]$, comparing this calculated pH (pH_c) to the measured pH (pH_m) tells whether there has been a movement of bicarbonate to protect (compensatory) or worsen (metabolic disorder) the pH. If the measured and calculated pH are within 0.03 unit, they are considered equal, and the acid–base disorder is acute or uncompensated. The use of the pH_c to identify the origin of acid–base imbalance from the ABG and to recognize mixed disorders is summarized

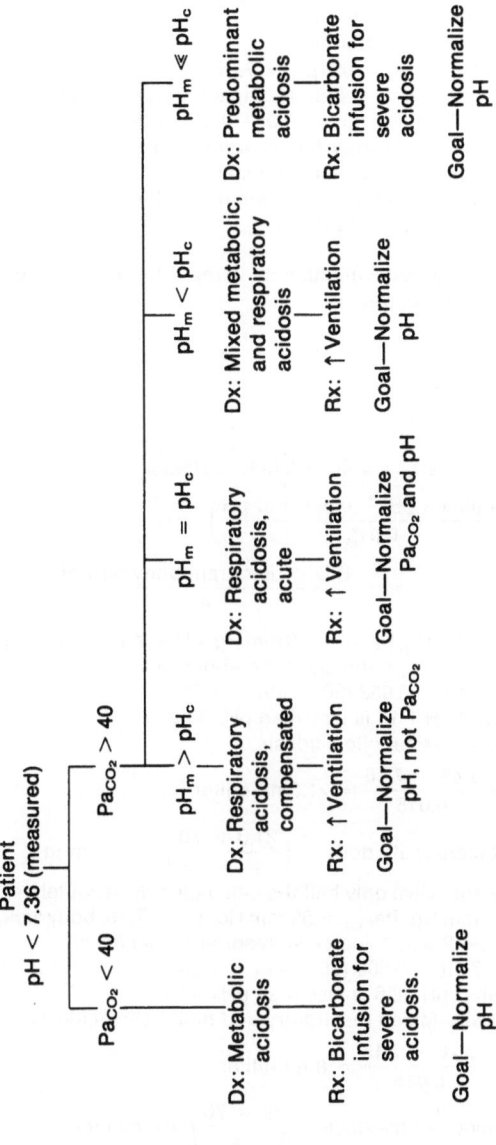

FIGURE 8. Using the ABG to evaluate and treat acidosis: the role of the calculated pH. pH_m = measured pH; pH_c = calculated pH = $7.40 - 0.008 \times (Pa_{CO_2} - 40)$ (see text); Dx = diagnosis; Rx = therapy.

Equation: $pH_c = 7.40 - 0.008 \ (Pa_{CO_2} - 40)$

Examples: 1. $Pa_{O_2} = 65$ mm Hg, $Pa_{CO_2} = 60$ mm Hg, pH = 7.24

    a. pH↓ and Pa_{CO_2} ↑ indicates respiratory acidosis.

    b. $pH_c = 7.40 - 0.008 \times (60 - 40) = 7.24$

    c. Measured pH (pH_m) 7.24 is equal to pH_c 7.24

    d. Diagnosis: Acute respiratory acidosis.

    e. Treatment: Increase ventilation with the goal of normalizing pH and Pa_{CO_2}.

    2. $Pa_{O_2} = 60$, $Pa_{CO_2} = 60$, pH = 7.34

    a. pH↓ and Pa_{CO_2} ↑ indicates respiratory acidosis.

    b. $pH_c = 7.40 - 0.008 \times (60 - 40) = 7.24$

    c. Measured pH (pH_m) 7.34 is greater than pH_c 7.24

    d. Diagnosis: Compensated respiratory acidosis.

    e. Treatment: Increase ventilation with the goal of normalizing pH, *not* Pa_{CO_2}.

FIGURE 9. Origin of the acid–base imbalance: using the calculated pH, pH_c. See text for explanation of the equation.

Equations: *Calculated* pH = $pH_c = 7.40 - 0.008 \times (Pa_{CO_2} - 40)$

$$B.D. = \left(\frac{\text{calculated pH} - \text{measured pH}}{0.015} \right)$$

$$\text{Total bicarbonate dose} = \frac{B.D. \times \text{kilogram body weight}}{4}$$

Examples: 1. $Pa_{O_2} = 100$ mm Hg, $Pa_{CO_2} = 30$ mm Hg, pH = 7.16, body weight = 70 kg

    a. pH↓ and Pa_{CO_2} ↓ indicates metabolic acidosis.

    b. $pH_c = 7.40 - 0.008 \cdot (30 - 40) = 7.48$

    c. Measured pH 7.16 is less than pH_c 7.48

    d. Diagnosis: Metabolic acidosis

    e. $B.D. = \dfrac{7.48 - 7.16}{0.015} = 21.3$ mEq/liter

    f. Total bicarbonate dose = $\left(\dfrac{21.3 \times 70}{4} \right) = 373$ mEq

    g. Treatment: Give only half the calculated dose acutely = 186.5 mEq

    2. $Pa_{O_2} = 55$ mm Hg, $Pa_{CO_2} = 55$ mm Hg, pH = 7.16, body weight = 70 kg

    a. pH↓ and Pa_{CO_2} ↑ indicates respiratory acidosis.

    b. $pH_c = 7.40 - 0.008 \cdot (55 - 40) = 7.28$

    c. Measured pH 7.16 is less than pH_c 7.28

    d. Diagnosis: Mixed respiratory and metabolic acidosis.

    e. $B.D. = \dfrac{7.28 - 7.16}{0.015} = 8$ mEq/liter

    f. Total bicarbonate dose = $\left(\dfrac{8 \times 70}{4} \right) = 140$ mEq

    g. Treatment: Since B.D. is small and bicarbonate infusion might exacerbate respiratory acidosis, treat by increasing ventilation and finding source of the metabolic acidosis.

FIGURE 10. Severe metabolic acidosis: using the base deficit (B.D.) for computation of bicarbonate dose.

in Fig. 8. Figure 9 illustrates the use of this formula in analyzing several cases.

The Calculated Base Deficit in the Treatment of Severe Acidosis

Although the ABG does not identify the source of metabolic impairment (e.g., renal, diabetic), it can be helpful in directing *acute therapy for severe metabolic acidosis*. In the emergency patient with acidosis, the ABG allows an approximation of the deficit of base or bicarbonate ion in the patient and hence the replacement dose of bicarbonate required for acute treatment. This *base deficit* (B.D.) is calculated by using another simple Henderson–Hasselbach-derived formula:

$$\text{B.D.} = \frac{(\text{pH}_c - \text{pH}_m)}{0.015}$$

(In this formula, 0.015 is the expected change in pH for each 1 mM/liter change in bicarbonate concentration at a constant Pa_{CO_2}.) The use of this formula to calculate B.D. and the dose of bicarbonate required for treatment is shown by examples in Fig. 10. The bicarbonate anion distributes itself acutely over extracellular fluid volume, which corresponds in approximate volume to 25% of ideal body weight.

OTHER CONSIDERATIONS IN ABG SAMPLING AND INTERPRETATION

When obtaining an ABG, the clinician wants to know the status of the gases and pH *in the patient*. If the sample is not correctly collected (anaerobically and with minimal heparin) and transported (sealed and iced), the ABG values measured will not reflect the in vivo conditions. See Table 2 for the effects on ABG measurement of excess heparin, air bubbles in the syringe, and failure to ice the specimen.

In addition, certain things about the patient strongly influence the ABG measurements. These must be known for an accurate interpretation of the results:

- Patient's *temperature*, febrile or hypothermic
- Patient's *body position*, upright or supine
- Any change in patient's *breathing pattern* during arterial puncture, hyperventilation or breath holding

TABLE 2. Considerations in Arterial Blood Gas Interpretation

	Effect on the ABG measurement		
1. The patient			
Position			
Seated	$\uparrow P_{O_2}$		
Supine	$\downarrow P_{O_2}$		
Anxiety			
Breath holding	$\downarrow P_{O_2}$,	$\uparrow P_{CO_2}$,	$\downarrow pH$
Hyperventilation	$\uparrow P_{O_2}$,	$\downarrow P_{CO_2}$,	$\uparrow pH$
Temperature			
Fever $\geq 104°F$	$\downarrow P_{O_2}$,	$\downarrow P_{CO_2}$,	$\uparrow pH$
Hypothermia $<94°F$	$\uparrow P_{O_2}$,	$\uparrow P_{CO_2}$,	$\downarrow pH$
2. The sampling technique (patient breathing room air)			
Quantity of heparin			
>0.1 cc/5 cc blood	$\uparrow P_{O_2}$,	$\downarrow P_{CO_2}$	
No heparin	Clotted specimen cannot be analyzed		
Large air bubbles	$\uparrow P_{O_2}$,	$\downarrow P_{CO_2}$,	$\uparrow pH$
Venous sample	$\downarrow P_{O_2}$,	$\uparrow P_{CO_2}$,	$\downarrow pH$
3. Sample transport and delay before analysis			
Temperature: room temperature	$\downarrow P_{O_2}$,	$\uparrow P_{CO_2}$,	$\downarrow pH$

- $F_{I_{O_2}}$
- *Mechanical ventilator settings:* rate, tidal volume, mode, positive end-expiratory pressure

The effects on the ABG measurement of some of these patient-determined factors are also summarized in Table 2.

In some situations it is difficult to tell whether the blood is being sampled from the artery or the vein; this usually occurs when the patient is in shock, with no palpable pulse. The alveolar air equation gives us a guideline for *recognizing an ABG measurement that is not venous.* The partial pressure of inspired oxygen [$P_{I_{O_2}}$ = (barometric pressure -47) $\times$ $F_{I_{O_2}}$] is approximately equal to the sum of P_{O_2} and P_{CO_2} in the alveolus. This $P_{I_{O_2}}$ is also the maximum pressure for the sum of P_{O_2} and P_{CO_2} in the capillary and artery. Hence, Pa_{O_2} + Pa_{CO_2} must be equal to or less than $P_{I_{O_2}}$. Since the normal arteriovenous difference is 45 for oxygen and 5 for carbon dioxide, one can calculate approximate arterial gas values from a venous measurement by adding 45 to P_{O_2} and subtracting 5 from P_{CO_2}. If the sum of these calculated arterial gases is greater than $P_{I_{O_2}}$, the original sample was probably arterial, not venous. If the sum of these calculated arterial gases is less than $P_{I_{O_2}}$, the original sample *may* have been arterial [with a large $P(A\text{-}a)_{O_2}$ or $P(a\text{-}v)_{O_2}$ present], or venous.

Whenever there is a question about the source of the blood (arterial or venous) for gas analysis, because of the finding of a low

Pa_{O_2} or high Pa_{CO_2}, another puncture must be made at a different arterial site and the blood sent for ABG analysis as soon as possible.

Complications of Arterial Puncture

The complications of arterial puncture include local infection, hematoma, occult bleeding, arterial thrombosis, ischemia of the distal extremity, and nerve trauma. The incidence of these complications is greatest for the femoral artery puncture. The preferred site of arterial puncture in descending order is radial, brachial, femoral. Complications are rare when the correct technique is used by an experienced practitioner with a small gauge needle.

SUMMARY

ABG analysis is useful in the emergency patient for defining blood oxygenation, identifying the probable cause of hypoxemia, defining the acid–base status of the patient, and identifying the probable cause of pH imbalance. Helpful computations using ABG values are given. Finally, other considerations that must be taken into account when interpreting the ABG are discussed and the complications of arterial puncture reviewed.

BIBLIOGRAPHY

1. Davenport HW: *ABC's of Acid Base Chemistry*. Chicago, University of Chicago Press, 1974.
2. Jones NL: *Blood Gases and Acid-Base Physiology*. New York, Thieme-Stratton, 1980.
3. Pontoppidan H: Acute respiratory failure in the adult (second part). *N Engl J Med* 287:743–752, 1972.
4. Snider GL: Interpretation of the arterial oxygen and carbon dioxide partial pressures. *Chest* 63:801–806, 1973.

PART II

Normal Lungs with Acute Respiratory Decompensation

CHAPTER 3

Extrapulmonic Ventilatory Failure

Ann Medinger

Ventilatory failure is a failure of the respiratory system to properly oxygenate and remove carbon dioxide from the blood. The respiratory system includes the pulmonary parenchyma (airways, alveoli, and capillary bed) and the pulmonary vessels; but it also includes the chest wall; the muscles of respiration; the nerves innervating the chest and diaphragm; the central and peripheral chemoreceptors; and the respiratory centers in the brain.

Patients having ventilatory failure due to pulmonic diseases (of the parenchyma or pulmonary vessels) must be distinguished from those with ventilatory failure due to extrapulmonic diseases (of chest wall, muscles, nerves, chemoreceptors, or brain) in order to give appropriate therapy.

The hallmark of *extra*pulmonic ventilatory failure (EPVF) is the maintenance of a normal gradient between alveolar and arterial oxygen tension $P(A-a)_{O_2}$, a value that is derived from the arterial blood gas (ABG) analysis. The ABG is a crucial element in identifying and treating EPVF.

DIFFERENTIAL DIAGNOSIS OF EXTRAPULMONIC VENTILATORY FAILURE

The differential diagnosis of diseases causing EPVF is divided into three physiologic categories:

Ann Medinger • Division of Pulmonary Diseases and Allergy, George Washington University School of Medicine and Health Sciences, Washington, D.C. 20037; Pulmonary Function Laboratory, Veterans Administration Medical Center, Washington, D.C. 20422.

- Decreased ventilatory drive
- Neural or muscular dysfunction
- Increased impedance

Category I: Decreased Ventilatory Drive

This category includes diseases in which the central control of respiration is impaired by sedation, infarction, or metabolic derangement. The most common cause of EPVF, an overdose of sedative drugs, is

TABLE 1. Extrapulmonic Ventilatory Failure (EPVF)—Category I.
Conditions Caused by Decreased Drive (P_{IMAX} = Normal)[a]

Disease	Incidence[b]	Diagnostic clue	Specific acute therapy[c]
Sedative overdose	F	Narcotic symptom complex: flaccid muscles; ↓ DTRs; slow pulse; cool skin; constricted, nonreactive pupils	For narcotics: naloxone
CNS medullary tumor	R	Ataxic breathing; may arrest without warning; no dyspnea sensation	
CNS medullary infarction	R	Ataxic breathing; may arrest without warning	
Myxedema	I	Hypothermia, "hung DTRs"	i.v. thyroxine
Severe metabolic alkalosis	I	History of loop diuretics	NH_4Cl or acetazolamide
Sleep apnea syndrome	I	Symptom complex: morning headache, loud snoring, daytime somnolence, hypertension, insomnia	
Primary hypoventilation	R	Apnea during sleep, normal awake breathing	
Multiple sclerosis	R	Cranial nerve dysfunction	
Encephalitis and postviral Reye's syndrome	I	Abnormal CSF (↑ serum NH_4^+ for Reye's)	Appropriate antibiotics; neurosurgical measures to normalize intracranial pressure

[a] DTR = deep tendon reflexes; i.v. = intravenous; CSF = cerebrospinal fluid; CNS = central nervous system; P_{IMAX} = maximal inspiratory pressure.
[b] Incidence among emergency room cases of EPVF: F = frequent; I = infrequent; R = rare.
[c] Temporary or permanent ventilatory support may be needed. See text heading Indications for Mechanical Ventilation.

Equipment:
- Manometer capable of measuring subatmospheric pressure and,
- Face mask or
- Mouthpiece and noseclip and
- Y connector

Method:

Awake patient:

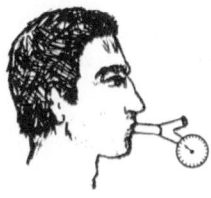

1. After explaining the procedure and asking permission, assemble the mouthpiece, Y connector, and manometer; stop the patient's nasal airflow with noseclips.
2. Instruct the patient to seal his lips around the mouthpiece and breathe through the apparatus.
3. Obstruct the airflow on inspiration by occluding the open arm of the Y connector, instructing the patient to sustain his best inspiratory effort for 10–15 sec.
4. Record the pressure that is sustained for 10 sec.
5. Repeat this measurement several times to obtain a consistent value.

Unconscious patient:

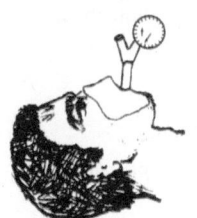

1. Connect the manometer to the mask by using the Y connector, and seal the mask tightly around the patient's nose and mouth. (Also works with endotracheal tube instead of a mask.)
2. Obstruct airflow on inspiration by occluding the open arm of the Y connector. Maintain this obstruction for 10–15 sec and record the patient's sustained inspiratory pressure.
3. Repeat the measurement several times to obtain a consistent value.

FIGURE 1. Measuring the maximum static inspiratory pressure (P_{Imax}).

included in this category. The differential diagnosis of other conditions in this category is listed in Table 1 along with diagnostic clues and specific therapies. The hallmark of this category of diseases is slow, quiet breathing. The static inspiratory pressure (P_{IMAX}) is normal, distinguishing this category of diseases from the next. P_{IMAX} is a simple bedside test described in Fig. 1. It can be measured whether the patient is unconscious or awake. If measured, the vital capacity and maximum breathing capacity are normal.

Category II: Neural or Muscular Dysfunction

This category of diseases of nerve, muscle, and neuromuscular junction includes infections involving the central nervous system and peripheral nerves, chemical toxins both synthetic and naturally occurring, metabolic disorders, and idiopathic diseases. The differential diagnosis, given in Table 2, lists diagnostic clues and specific therapies.

Amyotrophic lateral sclerosis, organophosphate poisoning, Guillain-Barré syndrome, and myasthenia gravis are the most common disorders

TABLE 2. Extrapulmonic Ventilatory Failure (EPVF)—Category II.
Conditions Caused by Neuromuscular Dysfunction ($P_{I_{MAX}}$ = Reduced)[a]

Diseases	Incidence[b]	Clinical clues	Specific acute therapy[c]
Corticospinal tracts and anterior horn cell			
Poliomyelitis	I	History of fever and muscle spasms; asymmetrical muscle weakness, absent DTRs	
Amyotrophic lateral sclerosis	I	Men 50–70 years; bilateral progressive weakness peripheral muscles, fasciculations	
Tetanus	I	Involuntary painful muscle spasms	Wound debridement, penicillin, human immune globulin
Traumatic cervical cordotomy	I	Trauma with acute quadriplegia	Immobilization of neck
Peripheral nerve			
Guillain-Barre syndrome	I	Progressive ascending motor weakness, absent DTRs	
Diphtheria	R	Recent history of severe skin infection or pharyngitis with pharyngeal membrane; associated with cranial nerve weakness	Penicillin and diphtheria antitoxin
Idiopathic or postzoster phrenic neuropathy	R	Supine dyspnea, normal upright; abdominal retraction on inspiration	Upright position
Porphyria	R	Young adult; associated abdominal pain; associated psychiatric or CNS signs; antecedent voice alteration; paradoxical diaphragmatic movement	Chlorpromazine may help
Neuromuscular junction			
Myasthenia gravis	I	History of fatigue; physical examination for ptosis and diplopia	Edrophonium
Cholinergic crisis	I	History of myasthenia on medication; history of abdominal pain, diarrhea; physical examination for fasciculations	Atropine
Organophosphate poisoning	I	History of crop picking in insecticide sprayed fields	Atropine and pralidoxine

TABLE 2. (*continued*)

Diseases	Incidence[b]	Clinical clues	Specific acute therapy[c]
Botulism	I	History of eating home-canned food; dizziness, dry mouth, facial nerve symptoms initially	Penicillin, polyvalent antitoxin
Succinylcholine (in patients with cholinesterase deficiency	I	History of succinylcholine therapy	
Aminoglycoside idiosyncratic reaction	R	History of aminoglycoside therapy	
Tick paralysis	I	Progressive motor weakness; southern and western U.S.	Find and remove tick
Muscle			
Muscular dystrophies	R	Symmetrical proximal weakness, DTRs normal	
Periodic paralysis		Familial; early-morning weakness; K^+ ↑, ↓, or normal	$[K^+]$ low: Potassium $[K^+]$ high: Glucose/insulin $[K^+]$ normal: NaCl
Inflammatory myopathy (polymyositis, dermatomyositis)	R	Muscles weak and tender	
Metabolic			
Hypercalcemia	R		NaCl/diuretics (calcitonin)
Hypophosphatemia	R		Phosphate
Hypokalemia	R		KCl
Hyperkalemia	R		Glucose/insulin
Rhabdomyolysis	R	Red urine, tender muscles	Diurese and alkalinize urine

[a] DTRs = deep tendon reflexes; CNS = central nervous system; P_{IMAX} = maximal inspiratory pressure.
[b] Incidence among emergency room cases of EPVF: F = frequent; I = infrequent; R = rare.
[c] Temporary or permanent ventilatory support may be needed. See section on Indications for Mechanical Ventilation.

in this category of conditions causing EPVF. All patients with diseases in this category breathe best sitting upright; this gives them the best mechanical advantage in breathing, since visceral organs hang away from the weak diaphragm. Many of these patients are agitated and struggling to breathe. They sense that they need to move more air, since central control mechanisms are intact, but their neuromuscular apparatus is unable to respond adequately.

The patient with these diseases has a low P_{IMAX}. If measured, the

TABLE 3. Extrapulmonic Ventilatory Failure (EPVF)—Category III:
Conditions Caused by Increased Impedance[a]

Disease	Incidence[b]	Clinical clue	Specific acute therapy[c]
Massive obesity	I	Wt (kg) > Ht (cm)	Upright position
Massive ascites	I	Tense, protuberant abdomen	Paracentesis
Third-trimester pregnancy	R	Large fetus in proportion to mother's height	Upright position
Kyphoscoliosis	I	Hunchback	
Ankylosing spondylitis	R	Lateral spine film— bamboo spine	
Chest trauma with pneumothorax or massive effusion	I	Chest x ray	Chest tube

[a] Wt = weight in kilograms; Ht = height in centimeters.
[b] Incidence among emergency room cases of EPVF: F = frequent; I = infrequent; R = rare.
[c] Temporary or permanent ventilatory support may be needed. See text heading Indications for Mechanical Ventilation.

vital capacity, tidal volume, and maximum breathing capacity are also reduced.

Category III: Increased Impedance

These conditions are all associated with stiffening or compression of the lungs in the thoracic cavity. This increases the inspiratory work of each ventilatory excursion and, hence, the work of achieving an adequate minute ventilation. The differential diagnosis of these conditions is given in Table 3 with diagnostic clues and specific therapies.

ABG IN DIAGNOSIS AND MANAGEMENT OF EPVF

Though signs and symptoms (discussed below) may suggest the general diagnosis of respiratory failure, the ABG clinches the diagnosis of EPVF:

- Pa_{O_2} is reduced (<75)
- Pa_{CO_2} is elevated (>50)
- $P(A-a)_{O_2}$ is normal (<25)

Importance of $P(A\text{-}a)_{O_2}$

An elevated $P(A\text{-}a)_{O_2}$ indicates concomitant and usually primary pulmonic disease. Hypercapneic respiratory failure is usually due to one of the following:

- Pulmonary airway diseases (chronic airway obstruction and acute severe asthma)
- Diseases causing EPVF (see Tables 1, 2, 3)

The $P(A\text{-}a)_{O_2}$ is always elevated (usually mildly, 25–50) in respiratory failure due to airway disease.

Computation of $P(A\text{-}a)_{O_2}$

$$P(A\text{-}a)_{O_2} = (P_B - 47) \times F_{I_{O_2}} - \frac{Pa_{CO_2}}{0.8} - Pa_{O_2}$$

Further discussion of the derivation and interpretation of the $P(A\text{-}a)_{O_2}$ is found in Chapter 2.

ABG Guidance in the Treatment of Acidosis

In the patient with EPVF, a pH less than 7.20 portends impending cardiovascular collapse. The appropriate urgent therapy is determined by the source of the acidosis, whether primarily respiratory or metabolic. (Severe acute respiratory acidosis may require immmediate endotracheal intubation and assisted ventilation. Severe metabolic acidosis may require intravenous bicarbonate therapy.) The primary source of the acidosis can be identified from the ABG by comparing the measured pH to the calculated pH:

- Measured pH $\geq$ calculated pH $\rightarrow$ predominant respiratory acidosis
- Measured pH $<$ calculated pH $\rightarrow$ mixed acidosis
- Measured pH $\ll$ calculated pH $\rightarrow$ predominant metabolic acidosis (difference $> 7.40 -$ calculated pH)

Computation of Calculated pH

$$\text{pH calculated} = 7.40 - 0.008 \times (Pa_{CO_2} - 40)$$

Further discussion of the derivation and uses of the calculated pH is found in Chapter 2.

Comment

Hypercapneic ventilatory failure that is acute and severe enough to cause even moderate respiratory acidosis (pH 7.20–7.30) on the initial ABG requires repeat ABG measurements during further diagnostic and therapeutic maneuvers until the patient is improved and stable. There are no sufficiently reliable clinical signs to replace repeated measurements of the ABG in assessing the patient's status and anticipating abrupt deterioration.

EMERGENCY EVALUATION OF THE PATIENT WITH EPVF

History

The patient with EPVF may have a chief complaint ranging from supine dyspnea (a sign of paresis of the diaphragm) or diffuse morning headaches to severe agitation, confusion, or coma (caused by the rising Pa_{CO_2}). The historical information that should be elicited includes drug use, symptoms of depression, antecedent neurologic problems, respiratory symptoms, and trauma. Historical clues that predispose the patient to extrapulmonic ventilatory failure include the following:

- Illicit i.v. or other drug use
- Depression with access to sedative medications
- Farm work picking fruits or vegetables in insecticide-sprayed fields
- Prior neuromuscular disease or weakness
- Hypertension with antecedent headache or neurologic symptoms
- Camping or working in tick-infested woods
- Progression of headache, drowsiness, stupor, or coma

Physical Examination

The physical examination should concentrate on vital signs, gross evidence of head trauma, level of consciousness, breathing rate and pattern, pupillary size and response, funduscopic examination, eye position and reflex movements, extremity motor function, pathologic movements or posturing, deep tendon reflexes, and pathologic reflexes. It is helpful to obtain $P_{I_{MAX}}$, if available (see Fig. 1).

Objective clues from the physical examination that suggest EPVF include the following:

- Quiet, shallow, slow, or irregular breathing

- Small pupils that react briskly to light
- Papilledema (occasionally)
- Asterixis and multifocal myoclonus
- Increased muscle tone
- Depressed deep tendon reflexes
- Extensor plantar reflexes
- When oxygen therapy has been given, flushed skin and low blood pressure may be present

Physical findings of acute or chronic lung disease (rales, rhonchi, wheezes, prolonged inspiration, hyperresonance, or dullness to percussion of the chest) make EPVF unlikely as a primary diagnosis.

Further clues from the physical examination that may point to the etiology of EPVF include

- Third-trimester pregnancy
- Massive obesity
- Massive ascites
- Needle tracks along peripheral veins
- Evidence of myxedema (coarse hair, very depressed or "hung" deep tendon reflexes, hypothermia, peripheral edema)
- Generalized bilateral motor weakness in an awake patient
- Signs of chest or head trauma
- Chest wall deformity
- Signs of a cerebrovascular accident (deep tendon reflex or motor asymmetry, asymmetry of pathologic reflexes, deviation of eyes)

Laboratory Assessment

The ABG analysis, discussed previously, confirms the diagnosis of EPVF. The inspiratory pressure ($P_{I_{MAX}}$), described in Fig. 1, is a simple bedside test that distinguishes between EPVF due to neuromuscular dysfunction and that due to central depression, as discussed previously. Other tests to help identify the specific diagnosis are listed in Tables 1, 2, and 3.

EMERGENCY MANAGEMENT OF EPVF

Before the results of ABG analysis are known, or a complete history and physical examination are obtained, the following general measures must be followed:

- If the patient is comatose, evaluate pulse, blood pressure and respiration, and initiate cardiopulmonary resuscitation if indicated.
- If the patient is stuporous or comatose and signs point to narcotic overdose, administer naloxone immediately, 0.4 mg i.v., i.m., or s.c., repeated every 2 min if necessary for a total of three doses. An awakening response to this therapy confirms the diagnosis of narcotic overdose. Repeat parenteral dosage of 0.4 mg. may be needed if signs of somnolence or respiratory depression recur.
- If the patient is agitated, confused, or comatose, and naloxone is not indicated or is unsuccessful, draw blood for ABG analysis and chemistry (blood urea nitrogen, electrolytes, blood sugar, and calcium) immediately, and initiate low-flow oxygen therapy (2 liters/min by nasal prongs or 28% by Venturi mask).
- If the patient is stuporous or comatose, respiratory rate is below 10, and naloxone is not indicated or unsuccessful, bag-mask ventilatory assistance must be given and arrangements made for endotracheal intubation.

Indications for Mechanical Ventilation in EPVF

Deciding when to initiate ventilatory assistance is a key therapeutic issue in managing patients with EPVF of any etiology. Most patients with EPVF never need mechanical ventilation. Many have chronic compensated conditions; others respond to therapeutic modalities, such as naloxone. However, in the acutely deteriorating patient (rising Pa_{CO_2}, falling pH), greatest success depends on initiating mechanical ventilation before cardiopulmonary collapse occurs. Often this must be done before a specific diagnosis can be reached.

Mechanical ventilation should be initiated in the following circumstances:

- After finding coma and shallow respirations under 10 per min on initial physical examination, and no indication for or success with naloxone therapy, initiate bag and mask ventilation and prepare for intubation and mechanical ventilation.
- After finding hypoxemia, hypercarbia, a normal $P(A-a)_{O_2}$, and a pH <7.20 with pure or primary respiratory acidosis (measured $\geq$ calculated pH) on the first ABG analysis, and no indication for or success with naloxone therapy, initate urgent intubation and mechanical ventilation to prevent cardiopulmonary collapse.
- Subsequent deterioration in either the patient's respiratory status and/or his arterial pH may require later intubation and assisted ventilation.

Complications of EPVF

The most serious complication of extrapulmonic failure is cardiorespiratory arrest. Frequent complications, occurring because the individual is unable to clear and defend his airways, include

- Aspiration pneumonia
- Bacterial pneumonia
- Segmental or lobar atelectasis from inspissated secretions

Other complications common to all patients with severe hypercapnia and/or hypoxia include

- Profound hypotension when high-flow oxygen is administered without improving ventilation (due to hypercapnia)

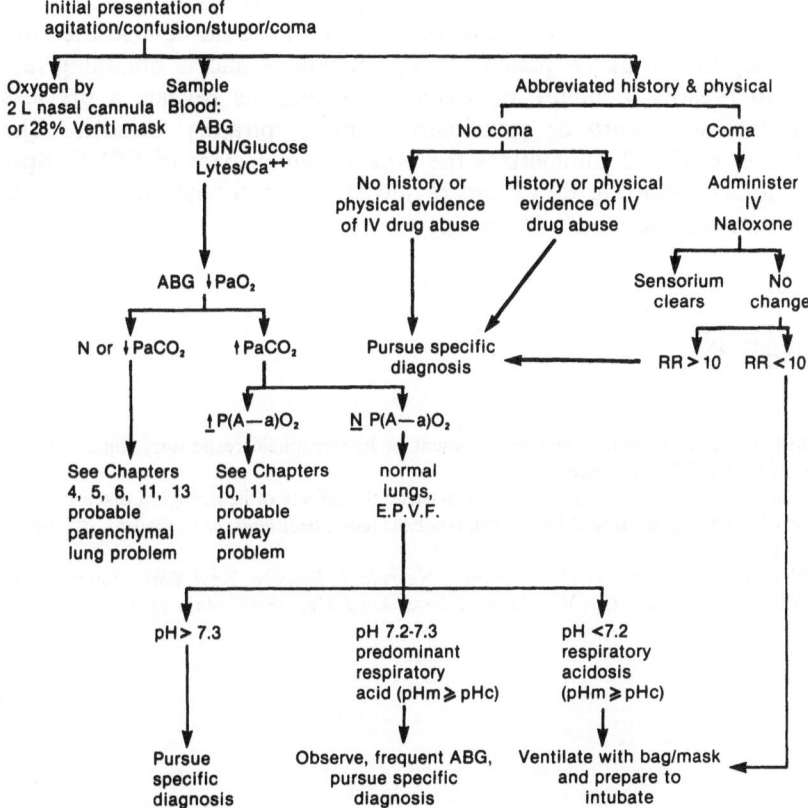

FIGURE 2. Algorithm for urgent management of extrapulmonic ventilatory failure. pHm, measured pH; pHc, calculated pH; $P(\text{A-a})_{O_2}$, alveolar-arterial oxygen difference; Lytes, serum electrolytes.

- Right-heart failure
- Left-heart failure
- Cardiac arrhythmias (due to hypoxemia)

When the degree of respiratory insufficiency requires mechanical ventilatory support, these patients are also subject to the complications that accompany the use of this modality. These are reviewed in Chapter 16.

SUMMARY

EPVF is associated with a low Pa_{O_2}, high Pa_{CO_2}, and normal $P(A-a)_{O_2}$ on ABG analysis. The major goals of emergency therapy are to improve oxygenation (increasing the Pa_{O_2}) and ventilation (improving the pH by lowering Pa_{CO_2}). Assisted ventilation should be instituted immediately in the EPVF patient who is comatose and is breathing less than 10 breaths a minute or when ABG analysis reveals a pH less than 7.20 with pure or principally acute respiratory acidosis. The algorithm in Fig. 2 summarizes the urgent management of EPVF. Specific diseases causing EPVF are reviewed with reference to diagnostic clues and specific modes of therapy.

BIBLIOGRAPHY

1. Kirk B: Early diagnosis and management of hypercapneic respiratory failure. *Semin Respir Med* 2:33–37, 1980.
2. Plum F: Breathlessness in neurologic disease; the effects of neurological disease on the act of breathing, in Howell JBL, Campbell EMJ (eds): *Breathlessness*. Oxford, Blackwell, 1966.
3. Weiner WJ: *Respiratory Dysfunction in Neurologic Disease*. New York, Futura, 1980.
4. Williams MH, Skim CS: Ventilatory failure. *Am J Med* 48:477–483, 1970.

CHAPTER 4

Life-Threatening Pneumonia

Morgan D. Delaney, Samuel V. Spagnolo, and Ann Medinger

Pneumonia is inflammation of the lung parenchyma. This chapter discusses only pneumonia due to infectious agents. See Chapter 5 for discussion of pneumonia due to the inhalation of pulmonary toxins.

Pneumonia becomes life-threatening when it seriously compromises gas exchange in the lung, causing acute respiratory failure. A number of factors may combine to increase the morbidity associated with infection of the lung parenchyma, including (1) virulence of the organism, (2) extent of infection, (3) failure of the patient to seek medical attention early in the illness, (4) abnormal host defenses, and (5) other underlying chronic disease states. The clinician's goal is, first, to recognize the presence of pneumonia and its severity, and then to identify the responsible microorganisms and institute specific antibiotics directed against them.

RECOGNIZING LIFE-THREATENING PNEUMONIA

The recognition of life-threatening pneumonia depends on a knowledge of

- The risk factors

Morgan D. Delaney • Pulmonary Laboratory, Division of Pulmonary Diseases and Allergy, George Washington University School of Medicine and Health Sciences, Washington, D.C. 20037.   Samuel V. Spagnolo • Division of Pulmonary Diseases and Allergy, Department of Medicine, George Washington University School of Medicine and Health Sciences, Washington, D.C. 20037; Pulmonary Disease Section, Veterans Administration Medical Center, Washington, D.C. 20422.   Ann Medinger • Division of Pulmonary Diseases and Allergy, George Washington University School of Medicine and Health Sciences, Washington, D.C. 20037; Pulmonary Function Laboratory, Veterans Administration Medical Center, Washington, D.C. 20422.

TABLE 1. Clinical Settings in Which Pneumonia May Be Life-Threatening

Old age	Asplenism
Debilitation or malnutrition	Sickle cell anemia
Chronic alcoholism	Immunocompromised host
Presence of chronic medical diseases	Chronic corticosteroid therapy
Chronic lung disease	Cancer
Congestive heart failure	Oncologic drug usage
Chronic renal disease	Disease that impairs the immune system
Diabetes mellitus	Neutropenia
Seizure disorder	Antecedent influenza
Prior stroke	

- The findings on history and physical examination
- The x ray and laboratory data

Pneumonia is likely to become severe and potentially life-threatening in a number of clinical settings listed in Table 1. Table 2 links frequently associated pathogens with common risk factors. Table 3 lists the physical findings that often accompany life-threatening pneumonia. Arterial blood gas (ABG) analysis should be performed in patients with pneumonia. Severe hypoxemia ($Pa_{O_2} < 60$ mm Hg) or an elevated Pa_{CO_2} with an accompanying respiratory acidosis indicates that there is a severe gas ex-

TABLE 2. Pneumonia Risk Factors and Associated Pathogens

Risk factor	Associated pathogens
Cigarette smoker with chronic obstructive lung disease	*Hemophilus influenzae* *Streptococcus pneumoniae*
Alcoholism	*Streptococcus pneumoniae* Anaerobic bacteria *Klebsiella pneumoniae* Staphylococci *Hemophilus influenzae*
Diabetes mellitus	Staphylococci Gram-negative bacteria *Mycobacterium tuberculosis* Mucormycosis
Multiple myeloma	*Streptococcus pneumoniae*
Sickle cell anemia	*Streptococcus pneumoniae*
Hospitalization	Gram-negative bacteria
Seizures, strokes	Anaerobic bacteria
Neutropenic states	Gram-negative bacteria, fungi, *Nocardia*
Immunologic deficiencies	*Pneumocystis carinii, Nocardia, Toxoplasma gondii,* fungi, mycobacteria
Gastrectomy	*Mycobacterium tuberculosis*
Silicosis	*Mycobacterium tuberculosis*
Prior viral infection	*Streptococcus pneumoniae* Staphylococci *Hemophilus influenzae*

TABLE 3. Identification of Severe Pneumonia from Clues Obtained by Physical Examination

Obvious respiratory distress
  Tachypnea
  Labored breathing
  Use of accessory muscles of respiration
Tachycardia
Hypotension
Abnormal mental status
  Confusion
  Obtundation
Signs of consolidation of an entire lung or involvement of both lungs
Signs of a pleural effusion
Signs of pulmonary hypertension or cor pulmonale
Cyanosis
Toxic-appearing patient [fever >102°F (adult)]
Hemoptysis
Evidence of extrapulmonary infection
  Pericarditis (friction rub)
  Endocarditis (murmur, embolic phenomena)
  Septic arthritis
  Meningitis (meningeal signs)
  Brain abscess (seizures, focal neurologic findings)

TABLE 4. Identification of Severe or Complicated Pneumonia from Clues Obtained by Chest X Ray

Total consolidation of more than one lobe	Diffuse interstitial infiltrates
Air fluid level, pneumatoceles, or cavitation	Bulging lobar fissure
	Large pleural effusion
Severe underlying parenchymal lung disease	Hilar mass
	Cardiomegaly

TABLE 5. Factors to Be Considered when Assessing the Severity of Pneumonia and Need for Hospitalization

History	Laboratory
Age <2 or >60 years	Pa_{O_2} <60 mm Hg
Poor general physical condition	Pa_{CO_2} >45 mm Hg
Chronic heart or lung disease	Leukopenia
Immunocompromised	Chest x ray
Abnormal mental status	Pleural effusion or extensive lung
Evidence of associated extrapulmonic	involvement
infection	Other
Physical examination	Suspicion of *Legionella*, staphylococcal,
Temperature >104°F (oral)	or gram-negative bacterial pneumonia
Blood pressure <100 mm Hg, systolic	
Pulse rate >120/min	
Respiratory rate >30/min	
Cyanosis	

change defect. Prompt intervention is required to assure adequate gas exchange. Chest x rays (posteroanterior and lateral) are needed to confirm the presence and extent of penumonia. Table 4 lists findings on the chest x ray that are associated with severe pneumonia and almost demand hospitalization. A complete blood count should be obtained; leukopenia suggests overwhelming infection.

Table 5 summarizes clinical factors that help determine the severity of the pneumonia and the need for hospitalization and intensive therapy.

IDENTIFICATION OF THE SPECIFIC PATHOGEN

Examination of Respiratory Tract Secretions

Careful microscopic examination of sputum [lower-respiratory-tract (LRT) secretions] is essential for determining the etiology of the pneumonia. Microscopic identification of the pathogen allows institution of specific antimicrobial therapy. The patient may be raising sputum spontaneously; if not, a variety of techniques are available to obtain diagnostic material:

- *Sputum induction* A heated aerosol of hypertonic saline is nebulized for at least 10–15 min to stimulate sputum production. (Occasionally, longer periods are required.)
- *Nasotracheal suctioning* A sterile, soft-rubber catheter (attached to a vacuum source with a collection trap in the line) is inserted through the nose into the trachea to aspirate tracheal secretions. This specimen is usually contaminated with mouth flora; this fact must be weighed when interpreting the gram stain and subsequent cultures of the aspirate.
- *Translaryngeal aspiration* A polyethylene catheter is inserted through a large needle that has punctured the cricothyroid membrane into the tracheal lumen; tracheal secretions are aspirated into a sterile syringe. A small amount of sterile saline solution may be instilled to stimulate cough. This method avoids oropharyngeal contamination of the specimen and hence yields a representative specimen of lower-airway pathogens. However, it must be performed by an experienced person to minimize the complications of peritracheal bleeding and compression, hemoptysis, and subcutaneous emphysema.
- *Fiberoptic bronchoscopy* A fiberoptic bronchoscope is passed through the upper airway (nose or mouth) into the trachea and bronchi; bronchial or alveolar secretions may be aspirated through the suction channel. Double-sheathed aspiration catheters should

TABLE 6. Microscopic Criteria of a Satisfactory
Sputum Sample

Less than 25 squamous epithelial cells per low-power field
Greater than 25 leukocytes per low-power field
Presence of alveolar macrophages
Presence of columnar ciliated bronchial epithelial cell

be used in collecting the specimen to reduce the incidence of oropharyngeal contamination. The procedure must be performed by
an experienced bronchoscopist.

- *Transthoracic needle aspiration* A small-gauge needle (23 gauge or
  smaller) is used to percutaneously puncture the affected lung and
  aspirate lung tissue. In a small percentage of patients, this procedure may be complicated by pneumothorax; it requires an experienced physician.

It is important to obtain a representative sample of LRT inflammatory
secretions. Table 6 defines an adequate LRT sputum specimen. Gram
stain of sputum is performed to identify the presence of gram-positive
and/or gram-negative organisms. A technically adequate gram stain will
stain the cytoplasm of neutrophils pink (gram-negative). Several fields
should be examined under low power of the microscope to choose a representative area for high-power analysis. When tuberculosis is suspected,
or when gram stain does not demonstrate bacteria, an acid-fast stain
should be performed on the sputum specimen. Additional special stains
are needed if fungal or other infections (*Legionella, Pneumocystis, Aspergillus*) are suspected as the cause of the pneumonia.

Sputum specimens should be submitted for appropriate cultures
promptly after collection and after smears have been made for microscopic examination. Table 7 lists pathogens that most commonly cause
life-threatening pneumonia.

TABLE 7. Microorganisms Commonly Causing Life-Threatening
Pneumonia

Bacteria	Fungi
Streptococcus	*Aspergillus*
Staphylococci	*Candida*
Klebsiella	Zygomycetes (mucormycosis)
Pseudomonas	*Cryptococcus*
Serratia	Protozoa
Escherichia coli	*Pneumocystis*
Hemophilus influenzae	*Toxoplasma*
Proteus	Viruses
Anaerobic bacteria	Cytomegalovirus
Legionella	Varicella zoster
Mycobacteria	Influenza

Additional Helpful Diagnostic Studies

- *A white blood cell count* (WBC) and differential may help distinguish bacterial from viral infection. Leukocytosis with a predominance of polymorphonuclear leukocytes is more characteristic of bacterial pneumonias. A normal WBC with lymphocytosis is more characteristic of viral and myocoplasmal infection.
- *Blood cultures* may isolate the pathogen.
- *Serologic studies on serum or sputum* may be helpful when the gram stain does not identify the pathogen and when an atypical organism is suspected. Cold agglutinins and specific complement-fixation antibody titers may identify *Myocoplasma* infection in the acute phase. Acute and convalescent viral and *Legionella* serologies are most helpful for retrospective diagnosis.
- *Bronchial washing and lung biopsy*. Certain acute pneumonias (e.g., *Pneumocystis carinii*, miliary tuberculosis, fungal) frequently cannot be diagnosed by either examination of respiratory tract secretions or serologic studies. In such instances bronchoscopic lavage or lung biopsy may be required. Biopsy may be performed transbronchially through the fiberoptic bronchoscope or at thoracotomy under general anesthesia. Fiberoptic bronchoscopy has a lower morbidity than thoracotomy; it has a high diagnostic yield. However, thoracotomy does yield a larger specimen of lung tissue; it is the preferred procedure when the patient is extremely hypoxemic, suffers a coagulopathy, or cannot cooperate with the breath holding required during transbronchial lung biopsy through a fiberoptic bronchoscope.
- *Thoracentesis*. When pleural fluid is present, it should be aspirated and analyzed for the presence of the pathogen and for the early identification of empyema. See Chapter 15 regarding pleural fluid analysis.

TREATMENT OF LIFE-THREATENING PNEUMONIA

General Measures

Both supportive and specific therapeutic measures must be promptly instituted after the diagnosis of severe pneumonia is established. The general approach is summarized in Table 8. The highest priority should be given to assuring adequate tissue oxygen delivery. The ABG measurement, which initially documents the degree of hypoxemia and adequacy of alveolar ventilation, must be repeated at periodic intervals until the patient is stable. The adequacy of tissue perfusion for delivery of

TABLE 8. Clinical Approach to the Treatment of the
Patient with Severe Pneumonia

Assure adequate oxygenation
    Supplemental O_2
Assure adequate ventilation
    Does the patient require intubation and mechanical ventilation?
Assure adequate tissue perfusion
    Hydration
Institute specific antibiotic therapy
    Identify the specific pathogen if possible
Assure adequate clearance of respiratory tract secretions
    Chest physiotherapy
    Bronchodilators
Treat specific complications
    Empyema
    Hemoptysis
    Shock
    Disseminated intravascular coagulation

---

oxygen is monitored by following the heart rate, blood pressure, and
mental status or urine flow.

Blood Pressure Support

If the patient is hypotensive, rapid repletion of intravascular volume
must be achieved by intravenous infusion of normal saline solution. Occasionally, dopamine or dobutamine may be required to improve tissue
perfusion. If signs of right-heart failure develop, management of the patient's fluid-volume status may require serial measurements of the pulmonary capillary wedge pressure with a Swan–Ganz catheter.

Supplemental Oxygen

Oxygen should be given by either nasal cannula or face mask at a
flowrate high enough to maintain a Pa_{O_2} of at least 65–70 mm Hg. There
is no need to raise the Pa_{O_2} to normal (90–100 mm Hg) or supranormal
(>100 mm Hg). The adequacy of oxygen therapy must be assessed by
repeat ABG analysis.

Hydration

A normovolemic state should be maintained. The most important
method of loosening and thinning tenacious respiratory tract secretions

is by maintenance of an adequate intravascular fluid volume. Most patients with severe pneumonia require placement of an intravenous catheter for delivery of physiologic fluids and antibiotics.

Mechanical Ventilation

Some patients with pneumonia cannot be adequately oxygenated by raising the inspired oxygen concentration (FI_{O_2}); they usually have a large intrapulmonary shunt. These patients may need intubation with mechanical ventilation and the use of positive end-expiratory pressure (PEEP) to achieve adequate oxygenation. See Chapter 16 for description of the use of mechanical ventilation and PEEP.

Specific Antimicrobial Therapy

The appropriate antibiotic(s) must be chosen to treat the specific or suspected pathogen. One of the major goals of the initial diagnostic evaluation of the patient with life-threatening pneumonia is identification of the specific pathogen through analysis of the clinical clues (e.g., risk factors, sputum examination). Figures 1, 2, and 3 display an algorithm for identification of the specific cause of pneumonia and choice of initial therapy. When a specific pathogen cannot be immediately identified, initial empiric therapy should be chosen for the patient with life-threatening pneumonia. Empiric antimicrobial therapy should be directed against the probable microorganism for the clinical setting (see following two sections).

Before choosing an antibiotic, ask the patient whether there is any known antibiotic hypersensitivity. Choose the most effective antibiotic with the lowest toxicity. Most hospitalized patients with life-threatening pneumonia should be started on parenteral antibiotics to assure rapid onset of action and therapeutic blood levels. Table 9 lists the preferred antimicrobial therapy for the common severe pneumonias; note that the doses given are for normal renal function. Many antibiotic doses must be reduced in treating patients with impaired renal function.

Empiric Antimicrobial Therapy

General guidelines can be established for empiric antibiotic use in several commonly encountered life-threatening situations when no predominant or specific organism can be discerned by *microscopic* evaluation

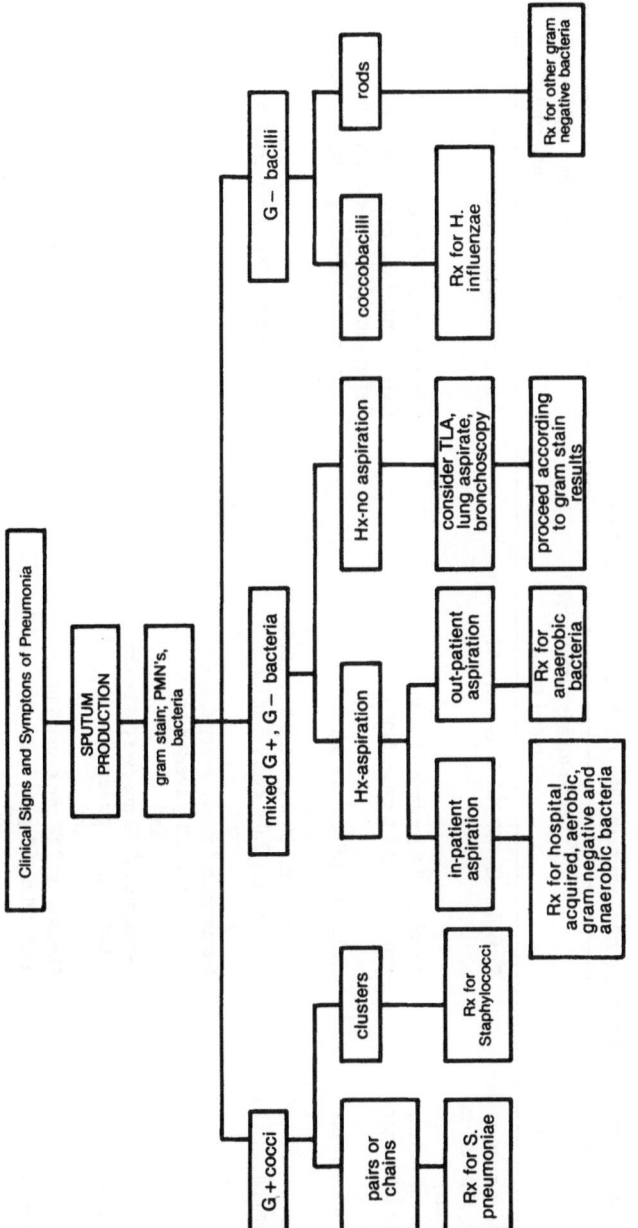

FIGURE 1. Algorithm for initial treatment of adults with pneumonia. G + = gram-positive bacteria; G − = gram-negative bacteria; PMNs = Polymorphonuclear white blood cells; TLA = translaryngeal aspirate; Hx = patient history; Rx = treatment. See also Figs. 2 and 3.

TABLE 9. Antimicrobial Therapy of Common Life-Threatening Pneumonias in Adults, 1985

Pathogen	Recommended treatment (dose and route[a])	Alternative regimen(s) (dose and route[a])
Streptococcus pneumoniae (formerly *Diplococcus pneumoniae*)	Penicillin G, 600,000 units every 12 hr i.m.	1 to 2 million units every 4 hr i.v.
Staphylococcus aureus	Nafcillin, 2.0 g every 4 hr i.v.	Vancomycin,[f] 500 mg every 6–8 hr i.v.
Hemophilus influenzae	Ampicillin, 2.0 g every 6 hr i.v.	Cefotaxime, 1.0 g every 6 hr i.v.
		Ceftazidime, 1.0–2.0 g every 8 hr i.v.
Klebsiella pneumoniae	Cefazolin, 1.0 g every 8 hr i.v. and	Ceftazidime, 1.0–2.0 g every 8 hr i.v.
	Gentamicin,[b] 80 mg every 8 hr i.m.	
Escherichia coli	Cefotaxime, 2.0 g every 8 hr i.v. and	Ceftazidime, 1.0–2.0 g every 8 hr i.v.
	Gentamicin,[b] 80 mg every 8 hr i.m.	
Proteus mirabilis	Cefotaxime, 2.0 g every 8 hr i.v. and	Ceftazidime, 1.0–2.0 g every 8 hr i.v. or
	Gentamicin,[b] 80 mg every 8 hr i.m.	Ampicillin, 2.0 g every 6 hr i.v.
Enterobacter sp.	Ticarcillin, 4.0 g every 6 hr i.v. and	Ceftazidime, 1.0–2.0 g every 8 hr i.v. or
	Gentamicin,[b] 80 mg every 8 hr i.m.	Gentamicin,[b] 80 mg every 8 hr i.m.
Serratia marcescens	Ticarcillin, 4.0 g every 6 hr i.v. and	Ceftazidime, 1.0–2.0 g every 8 hr i.v. and
	Gentamicin,[b] 80 mg every 8 hr i.m.	Tobramycin,[b] 80 mg every 8 hr i.m.

Organism		
Pseudomonas aeruginosa	Ticarcillin, 4.0 g every 6 hr i.v. and Tobramycin,[b] 80 mg every 8 hr i.m.	Ceftazidime, 2.0 g every 8 hr i.v. and Tobramycin,[b] 80 mg every 8 hr i.m.
Legionella sp.	Erythromycin, 0.5–1.0 g every 6 hr i.v.	Erythromycin, 1.0 g every 6 hr i.v. and Rifampin,[c] 600–900 mg once daily p.o.
Anaerobic bacteria *Peptostreptococcus* sp. *Peptococcus* sp. *Bacteroides* sp. *Fusobacterium* sp. *Propionibacterium* *Eubacterium* *Actinomyces* Microaerophilic streptococci	Clindamycin, 600 mg every 8 hr i.v.	Penicillin G, 600,000 units every 8 hr i.m. or 2.5 million units every 6 hr i.v.
Mycobacterium tuberculosis	Isoniazid, 300 mg daily[d] and Rifampin, 600 mg daily[d]	
Pneumocystis carinii	Trimethoprim, 15 mg/kg and Sulfamethoxazole, 75 mg/kg[e]	Pentamidine isethionate, 4.0 mg/kg i.m. or i.v. daily

[a] Doses are given for patients with normal renal function.
[b] Amikacin, 500 mg every 12 hr, may be substituted for gentamicin- or tobramycin-resistant isolates.
[c] Rifampin not to be used as a sole agent.
[d] Streptomycin, 0.75 mg to 1.0 g daily, and Ethambutol, 15 to 25 mg/kg, may be added to the regimen for critically ill patients.
[e] Total daily dose is divided into four equally divided doses.
[f] For use in treatment of methicillin-resistant staphylococci and/or where penicillin allergy is present.

of sputum. *Empiric therapy should never be instituted without antecedent complete evaluation of respiratory tract secretions and blood to identify the offending pathogen.*

General Guidelines for Empiric Therapy

- *Normal host, community-acquired infection.* The previously healthy patient, who has not been recently hospitalized, has no recognized risk factors for pneumonia such as underlying chronic disease, and fails to produce purulent sputum or provide gram stain identification of an organism from any LRT specimen, is likely to have pneumonia due to *Mycoplasma*, influenza virus, or *Legionella* species. There is no antibiotic of proven effectiveness against influenza virus; therefore, erythromycin should be chosen to treat possible *Mycoplasma* or *Legionella* infection.

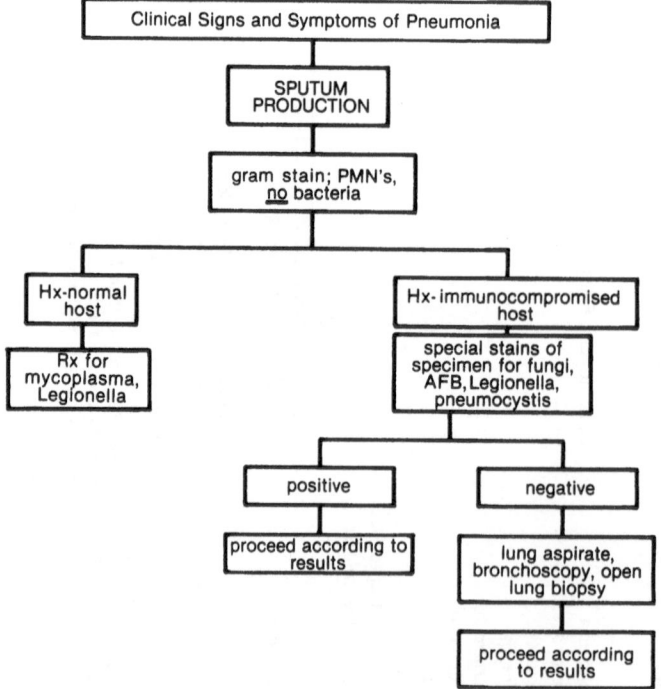

FIGURE 2. Algorithm for initial treatment of adults with pneumonia. G + = gram-positive bacteria; G – = gram-negative bacteria; PMNs = polymorphonuclear white blood cells; TLA = translaryngeal aspirate; Hx = patient history; Rx = treatment.

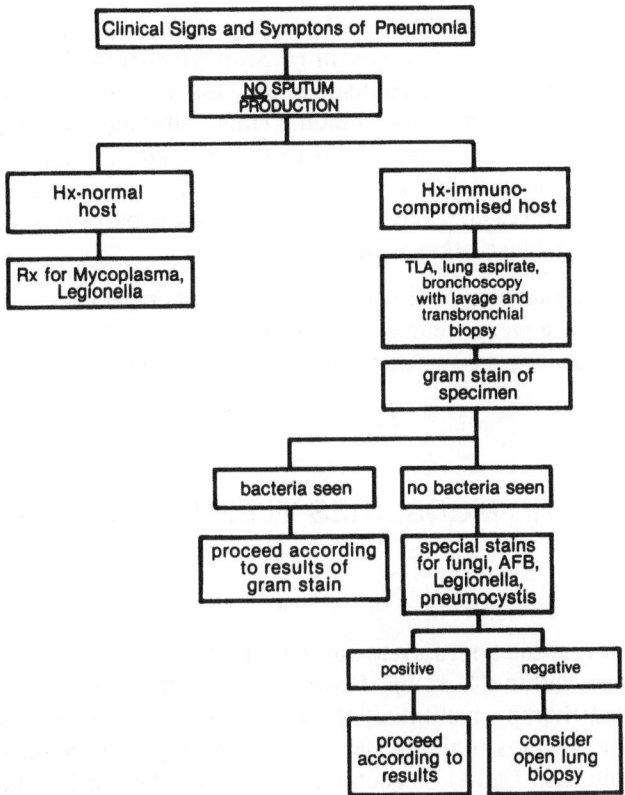

FIGURE 3. Algorithm for initial treatment of adults with pneumonia and no sputum production. G+ = gram-positive bacteria; G− = gram-negative bacteria; PMNs = polymorphonuclear white blood cells; TLA = translaryngeal aspirate; Hx = patient history; Rx = treatment.

- *Normal host, hospital-acquired infection.* The hospitalized patient who develops severe pneumonia frequently also has chronic medical problems. If not immunocompromised (not receiving corticosteroids, antineoplastic drug therapy, and having no known disease that has impaired the immune system), he is likely to have pneumonia due to a gram-negative bacteria (*Klebsiella pneumoniae, Enterobacter* sp., *Proteus* sp, *Serratia marcescens, Pseudomonas* sp., *Acinetobacter, Escherichia coli*) or due to staphylococcal infection. Hence, initial broad-spectrum antibiotic coverage should be given, usually including an aminoglycoside and either a penicillin derivative or a cephalosporin. This therapy should be continued until there is identification of a specific pathogen by culture.
- *Immunocompromised host.* The immunocompromised patient with neutropenia (WBC < 500) who develops clinical or roentgeno-

graphic findings of acute pneumonia is also likely to be infected with a gram-negative organism or *Staphylococcus*. However, infection with other opportunistic organisms (fungus, *Pneumocystis*, myobacteria) is not uncommon. Thus, although these patients should be given empiric broad-spectrum (usually a cephalosporin plus an aminoglycoside) antibiotic therapy, an aggressive diagnostic evaluation (which may include an open-lung biopsy) is important to look for these other pathogens.

The risks of inappropriate empiric antibiotic therapy include not only the possibility of adverse reactions to the drugs themselves, but also the emergence of pathogens resistant to the antimicrobials that have been administered.

OTHER THERAPEUTIC MODALITIES IN SEVERE PNEUMONIA

Antipyretics

Institution of the appropriate antimicrobial therapy usually results in defervescence within 24–48 hr. However, once the infection has been identified and therapy instituted, the patient may be treated with antipyretics if he remains toxic or symptomatic during fever spikes. Either acetylsalicylic acid (ASA) or acetaminophen may be used. (Check first for a prior history of allergy to ASA or acetaminophen.) Beware the use of antipyretics in patients receiving empiric therapy, because the response of the temperature curve may be an important piece of information.

Analgesics

These may be warranted if pleuritic chest pain is present. ASA or acetaminophen will usually suffice. Narcotic analgesics are occasionally necessary to control severe chest pain. Narcotics are relatively contraindicated when the respiratory center is depressed or the Pa_{CO_2} elevated. Beware using analgesics alone for pain that develops after the initial presentation; this often signifies pleural extension and demands further diagnostic assessment.

Bronchodilators

Aerosol β-adrenergic bronchodilators or parenteral aminophylline may be used in the patient with pneumonia who has acute bronchospasm or chronic airflow obstruction. Dosages are the same as used in acute asthma. (See Chapter 11.)

Antitussives

Cough is a physiologic mechanism for clearing obstructed airways. In treating pneumonia, the cough should be suppressed only when it is dry and profoundly irritative or when it prevents sleep. Codeine (10–30 mg) is the drug of choice for cough suppression; terpin hydrate and dextromethorphan may have some efficacy.

Other Measures

Stimulation of cough by nasotracheal suctioning may help some patients to clear their secretions. Bland aerosols and mucolytic agents delivered by aerosol have no proven value and may be detrimental, inducing bronchoconstriction in patients with reactive airways. If the clinical examination of the initial chest x ray suggests that an endobronchial foreign body or tumor is obstructing the airway, bronchoscopy is needed for diagnosis. The development of lobar collapse without air bronchograms on chest x ray indicates that a central airway is obstructed by inflammatory secretions; chest physiotherapy should be initiated to clear the obstructed bronchus. If physiotherapy fails to remove obstructing secretions, fiberoptic bronchoscopy may be needed.

SPECIFIC PNEUMONIAS

Streptococcus pneumoniae

This is the most common cause of bacterial pneumonia, particularly community-acquired. It can occur in previously healthy individuals as well as in those with chronic cardiac or pulmonary disease, diabetes mellitus, alcoholism, cirrhosis, or compromised immunity. The classical presentation includes a shaking chill, preceding high fever, cough, and purulent sputum production. Lobar or segmental consolidation is seen on the chest x ray; cavitation is rare. Gram stain of the sputum demonstrates many gram-positive diplococci, but it may be difficult to grow the organism on culture. Counterimmunoelectrophoresis may be used to detect the bacterial antigen in serum. Penicillin is the drug of choice for therapy.

Erythromycin is used in the penicillin-allergic patient. Vancomycin is the drug of choice for the rare penicillin-resistant pneumococcus. (See Table 9 for dosage.) Parapneumonic effusions are common (>50% of patients). The pleural fluid should be sampled by thoracentesis to rule out empyema. If antibiotics are instituted early, the parapneumonic effusions rarely progress to empyema, requiring aggressive drainage. For discussion of the recognition and management of empyema, see Chapter 15.

Staphylococcal Pneumonia

This is seen most commonly in the newborn, the elderly, and in individuals who have had a viral respiratory tract infection. Chills, fever, cough, and purulent sputum are common. The patient appears very toxic. Chest x ray reveals either lobar consolidation or patchy infiltrates, and cavitation is common. Gram stain and culture of sputum are the most useful diagnostic tests. Gram stain of sputum should demonstrate numerous gram-positive cocci in clusters. Therapy consists of a penicillinase-resistant penicillin, such as nafcillin; a cephalosporin may be used cautiously in the patient allergic to penicillin. (See Table 9 for dosage.) Mortality is high even with early diagnosis and therapy.

Klebsiella pneumoniae

This is most often seen in alcoholics and in those with severe heart disease, lung disease, or diabetes mellitus. Symptoms begin abruptly. Fever is usually above 103°F. Typically, the sputum is brick-red or resembles currant jelly. The initial chest x ray may slow lobar consolidation, but multiple small cavities (radiolucent areas within the consolidation) often appear on subsequent chest x rays. Initial antimicrobial treatment should include a cephalosporin plus an aminoglycoside. (See Table 9 for dosage.)

Hemophilis influenzae

This is most often seen in children younger than 10 years of age or in adults with chronic bronchopulmonary disease or alcoholism. Symptoms include fever, chills, cough, and purulent sputum production, often preceded by upper-respiratory-tract symptoms. The chest film may show focal lobar densities or patchy infiltrates in several areas. Pleural effusions are frequently seen. Diagnosis can be made from gram stain of sputum showing small, pleomorphic, gram-negative coccobacillary forms. Culture may be difficult owing to the organism's fastidious growth requirements. Therapy consists of either ampicillin or a cephalosporin such as cefotaxime. (See Table 9 for dosage.) Response to therapy is related to the extent of underlying disease.

Other Gram-Negative Bacteria

These bacteria are likely to cause pneumonia in chronically or severely ill patients who are hospitalized, or in myelosuppressed/immunosuppressed patients. Fever, chills, cough, and purulent sputum production are usually present. The chest x-ray pattern is variable, but multiple radiolucencies within consolidated areas due to lung necrosis are common. The specific agent can often be identified in the gram stain of the sputum, but only the sputum culture is definitive. Initial therapy should include two broad-spectrum agents (usually an aminoglycoside and a cephalosporin), but it will vary with the local antimicrobial susceptibility patterns. (See Table 9 for dosage.)

Legionella

Legionella bacteria are gram-negative bacilli that cannot be seen on simple gram stain of sputum. Unlike other gram-negative pneumonias, the clinical course of legionnaires' disease may initially resemble a viral or mycoplasmal infection. The cough is usually dry and irritating. Diarrhea and central nervous system symptoms may be present. The chest x-ray abnormalities often progress rapidly from patchy infiltrates to bilateral lobar or whole-lung consolidation. Pleural effusions are common. Rapid diagnosis of *Legionella* pneumonia can be made by direct fluorescent antibody staining of tissue or respiratory tract secretions. Special culture media are required for growth of the bacteria. Erythromycin is currently the antibiotic of choice. Rifampin is extremely active against *Legionella* species in vitro and in animal models, but because of the possibility of rapid development of rifampin resistance, it should not be used as the sole agent in the treatment of *Legionella* infection. (See Table 9 for dosage.)

Anaerobic Bacteria

Pneumonia caused by anaerobic bacteria is seen most often in patients with gingival disease who also have a history of an altered state of consciousness, drug or alcohol abuse, and/or a seizure disorder, which predispose to aspiration of oropharyngeal secretions or gastric contents. Acute aspiration of liquid gastric contents may cause acute chemical injury to the lung with resultant adult respiratory distress syndrome with clinical, pathologic, and pathophysiologic features typical of that condition (see Chapter 6). Secondary pneumonia is a common complication of gastric aspiration; it is usually due to anaerobic bacteria if the aspiration occurred outside of the hospital.

Aspiration of oropharyngeal secretions usually leads to a subacute clinical presentation, with anaerobic pneumonia and abscess formation. Sputum is frequently, but not always, foul smelling. Cavitation on chest roentgenogram is usually present when the patient is first examined. Necrosis of lung may lead to hemoptysis. LRT secretions for culture must be collected *anaerobically* from below the larnyx. However, often this diagnosis is made on the grounds of clinical and x-ray evidence, supported by response to therapy, without cultural confirmation. Therapy includes either penicillin or clindamycin. (See Table 9 for dosages.)

Mycobacteria

The patient with miliary tuberculosis is usually ill with high fever, chilliness, weakness, and prostration. However, the onset of symptoms is usually gradual. The chest x ray reveals diffuse interstitial infiltrates with a minute (1–2 mm) nodular pattern. Sputum is usually lacking, and acid fast bacillus (AFB) smears are frequently negative. Caseating granulomas can be identified on tissue biopsy. Bone marrow or liver is commonly biopsied, but transbronchial lung biopsy is the best source of tissue. Initial treatment should include isoniazid (INH), rifampin, and ethambutol. If parenteral therapy is necessary, INH and streptomycin may be given initially.

Pneumocystis

Pneumonia due to *Pneumocystis* occurs in patients with depressed T-lymphocyte function. Patients at risk for the disease include organ transplant recipients, patients with malignancies and collagen–vascular disease who receive corticosteroids, and recently patients with the acquired immune deficiency syndrome (AIDS). In all groups, except the patients with AIDS, the onset of disease is usually abrupt with high fever, marked dyspnea, and dry cough; the clinical presentation in the AIDS patient may be more insidious and subacute. The chest x ray reveals a diffuse interstitial infiltrate. The organism must be identified either in respiratory tract secretions obtained by bronchoscopic lavage or percutaneous lung aspirate, or in lung tissue from transbronchial biopsy or open-lung biopsy.

The drug combination of trimethoprim–sulfamethoxazole has proven effective in both the treatment and prevention of the disease. Pentamidine isethionate is an alternative therapeutic agent.

BIBLIOGRAPHY

1. Bartlett JG, Finegold SM: Anaerobic infections of the lung and pleural space. *Am Rev Respir Dis* 110:56–77, 1974.
2. Edelstein PH, Meyer RD: Legionnaires disease: A review. *Chest* 85:114–120, 1984.
3. Ferstenfeld JE, Schlueter DP, Rytel, MW, et al: Recognition and treatment of adult respiratory distress syndrome secondary to viral interstitial pneumonia. *Am J Med* 58:709–718, 1975.
4. Holt S, Ryan WF, Epstein EJ: Severe *Mycoplasma pneumoniae. Thorax* 32:112–115, 1977.
5. Hughes WT: *Pneumocystis carinii* pneumonitis. *Chest* 85:810–813, 1984.
6. Levison ME, Mangura CT, Lorber B, et al: Penicillin versus clindamycin for the treatment of anaerobic lung abscess. *Ann Intern Med* 98:466–471, 1983.
7. Matthay RA, Greene WH: Pulmonary infections in the immunocompromised patient. *Med Clin North Am* 64:529–551, 1980.
8. Matthay RA, Moritz ED: Invasive procedures for diagnosing pulmonary infection: A critical review, in Reynolds HY (ed): *Clinics in Chest Medicine,* Vol 2. Philadelphia, WB Saunders, 1981, pp 3–18.
9. Murray BE, Moellering RC: Antimicrobial agents in pulmonary infections. *Med Clin North Am* 64:319–342, 1980.
10. Pierce AK, Sanford JP: Aerobic gram-negative bacillary pneumonias. *Am Rev Respir Dis* 110:647–658, 1974.
11. Spagnolo SV, Raver JM: Nine-month chemotherapy for pulmonary tuberculosis. *South Med J* 75:134–138, 1982.
12. Tuazon CU: Gram-positive pneumonias. *Med Clin North Am* 64:343–361, 1980.

CHAPTER 5

Acute Inhalation Lung Disease

Philip Witorsch and Sorell L. Schwartz

INTRODUCTION

A vast number of chemicals may cause acute injury and disease when inhaled. This may be the result of direct injury to the respiratory tract or secondary to the accumulation of toxic levels in the blood after absorption through the respiratory portal of entry. Such chemicals are encountered in a wide variety of occupational, avocational, and accidental settings (Table 1). Any acute injury or disease produced will be determined by the specific chemical properties of the gas or combination of gases inhaled, the presence or absence of particulate materials, the concentration of the toxic substances(s), the conditions of exposure, and the presence of underlying conditions in the exposed individual.

The physical state and physical characteristics of inhaled substances are important factors determining the nature and degree of toxicity that occurs. Various chemicals occur as fumes, gases, vapors, smoke, or dust; some exist in more than one of these physical states. The depth to which aerosols penetrate into the lung depends on particle size, density, shape, and aerodynamic properties, as well as the depth of respiration. Potentially harmful inhaled substances vary in size from just small enough to enter the upper respiratory tract down to gas molecules that may readily penetrate to the alveoli.

The site of respiratory damage is determined by the solubility of irritant gases; more soluble gases (e.g., chlorine, ammonia) predominantly

Philip Witorsch • Respiratory Care, Division of Pulmonary Diseases and Allergy, George Washington University School of Medicine and Health Sciences, Washington, D.C. 20037; Georgetown University Schools of Medicine and Dentistry, Washington, D.C. 20007; Center for Environmental Health and Human Toxicology, Washington, D.C. 20007. Sorell L. Schwartz • Georgetown University Schools of Medicine and Dentistry, Washington, D.C. 20007; Center for Environmental Health and Human Toxicology, Washington, D.C. 20007.

TABLE 1. Toxic Fumes and Gases—Sources, Characteristics, Acute Effects[a]

Substance	Source	Predominant effects	Comments
Acetaldehyde	Manufacture of chemicals, resins, plastics, rubber; domestic or commercial disinfectant use	Eye and upper respiratory irritation (low concentrations); respiratory depression and ARDS (high concentrations)	Direct irritant and CNS depressant; systemic effects
Acrolein	Manufacture of textiles, plastics, synthetic fiber, pharmaceuticals, soap, linseed oil	Intense eye and upper-respiratory irritation	
Ammonia	Manufacture of fertilizer, explosives, plastics, pharmaceuticals, chemicals, refrigerants; oil refining; furnace additives; accidents involving storage and transport	Immediate eye, upper-respiratory, skin irritation; laryngeal edema and/or ARDS with prolonged exposure and/or very high concentrations	Very highly soluble
Cadmium oxide	Ore smelting, welding, electroplating, brazing, soldering, ceramics, manufacture of engine bearings, batteries, paints, glass, plastics	Direct irritant and systemic effects; early upper respiratory irritation, fever, myalgia; later tracheobronchitis, ARDS, nephrotoxicity, hepatotoxicity	Systemic absorption via respiratory tract; biphasic illness
Carbon monoxide	Fires; exhaust fumes; household gas	Tissue hypoxia	No direct irritant effects; systemic effects
Chlorine	Manufacture of paper, textiles, pharmaceuticals, plastics; swimming-pool use; accidents involving storage or transport; mixing chlorine bleach with an acid cleaner	Early eye and upper-respiratory irritation; ARDS with prolonged exposure and/or very high concentrations	Highly soluble
Chromate	Ore smelting; electroplating	Tracheobronchitis; pneumonitis; nasal septal perforation	
Hydrogen chloride	Manufacture of dye, fertilizer, textiles, rubber; ore refining, welding; fires	Intense eye and upper-respiratory irritation	

TABLE 1. (*continued*)

Substance	Source	Predominant effects	Comments
Hydrogen fluoride	Metal refining; glass etching; welding; chemical industry	Intense eye and upper-respiratory irritation; later ARDS and pneumonia	
Hydrogen sulfide	Manufacture of chemicals, dye, rayon, rubber, fish meal; tanning; waste disposal; sewage; petroleum refining; volcanic activity	Upper- and lower-respiratory irritation, including ARDS with lower concentrations; respiratory depression with high concentrations	CNS depressant; offensive odor
Mercury vapor	Electrolysis; metallurgy; electrical industry; manufacture of chemicals, pharmaceuticals, thermometers; dental laboratories	Tracheobronchitis and ARDS; myoneural toxicity	
Metal fumes (zinc, copper, magnesium, aluminum, iron, manganese, nickel)	Welding; galvanizing; ore smelting, metal, shipyard and foundry work; sculpting; manufacture of alloys and permanganate	Metal fume fever (see text)	
Nitrogen dioxide	Farming (silo-filler's disease); electroplating; welding; combustion of cellulose film, guncotton, cordite, shoe polish; explosives manufacture and detonation; mining; missile and jet fuels; diesel engine exhaust; engraving; metal cleaning; industrial use of nitric acid; anesthesia	Bronchitis, bronchospasm, and ARDS; methemoglobinemia	Low solubility; latent period; triphasic illness (see text)
Ozone	Arc welding; flour bleaching; copy equipment; air pollution	Eye and upper-respiratory irritation; ARDS	
Phosgene (carbonyl chloride)	Metallurgy; manufacture of chemicals, dyes; welding; paint remover; fire fighting	ARDS	Latent period

(*continued*)

TABLE 1. (*continued*)

Substance	Source	Predominant effects	Comments
Phosphine (hydrogen phosphide)	Manufacture of chemicals, acetylene, insecticide, fireworks; welding; rustproofing; storage of aluminum phosphate	ARDS	
Pyrolysis products of Teflon	Teflon manufacture and use	Polymer fume fever (see text)	
Smoke	Fires	Upper-respiratory irritation; upper-airway obstruction; lower-airway obstruction; ARDS; CO poisoning; secondary bronchopulmonary infection	Variable effects depending on smoke constituents
Sulfur dioxide	Manufacture of paper, bleach, chemicals; refrigerants; preservatives; fumigants; petroleum refining; ore smelting	Eye and upper-respiratory irritation; laryngeal edema; ARDS	
Vanadium pentoxide, nickel carbonyl, selenium compounds, titanium tetrachloride, zirconium	Chemical industry	Bronchitis; ARDS	
Volatile chlorinated and fluorinated hydrocarbons	Glue sniffing; inhalation of freon propellants, cements, lacquers, paints, fingernail polish remover, lighter fluid, gasoline, antifreeze	Cardiac conduction defects and arrhythmias, central nervous system effects	Systemic extrapulmonary effects; no direct respiratory irritation

[a] CNS = central nervous system.

injure the upper respiratory tract, and more insoluble gases (e.g., nitrogen dioxide) have a greater propensity for lower-respiratory-tract injury (Table 1). Highly soluble gases, which produce immediate and often intense eye and upper-respiratory irritation, cause the exposed individual to leave the area of exposure promptly, thus limiting the extent of any lower-respiratory injury. When the exposed individual is unable to leave the area of exposure or when the concentration of the gas is very high, lower-respiratory injury may result as well.

While most inhaled toxic gases cause acute respiratory injury by direct irritation, in some cases (e.g., hydrogen sulfide), the inhaled gas is a central nervous system respiratory depressant as well as an irritant, and respiratory dysfunction may result from both direct irritation and central hypoventilation.

Most patients who sustain inhalational respiratory tract injury recover completely. Limited available studies do not show chronic residual pulmonary dysfunction following inhalation lung injury in most patients, but such effects may occur in some individuals.

GENERAL APPROACH TO POSSIBLE ACUTE INHALATION LUNG DISEASE

In most cases, the patient with an acute inhalational respiratory injury comes to medical attention because of his exposure, often in an occupational setting (Table 1). In such situations, the nature of the exposure (i.e., the chemicals involved and the conditions of exposure) can usually be determined by questioning the patient and/or witnesses, co-workers, or family members. This information is extremely important and should be determined as soon as possible, as it will often be critical to the subsequent management of the patient. This is especially pertinent for substances whose toxic effects may be delayed for a period of time [e.g., smoke, cadmium oxide, nitrogen dioxide (NO_2)], because the patient may initially appear well or have minimal symptoms, only to later deteriorate.

Occasionally, the exposure may not be readily evident. In patients presenting with otherwise unexplained symptomatology that could be the result of inhalation of toxic substances, a careful history of possible exposures should be obtained from the patient and/or any family members, co-workers, or other witnesses who may be available. Signs and symptoms that suggest the possibility of acute inhalation of toxic materials include altered mental state; neurologic manifestations; pulmonary edema; dyspnea; eye irritation; nose, mouth, or throat irritation; laryngeal edema; facial skin irritation; epistaxis; nausea, vomiting, and diarrhea; and bleeding diathesis.

Initial evaluation of patients with known or possible acute inhalational injury is outlined in Table 2. Any urgent, potentially life-threatening problems should be dealt with immediately, even before the initial evaluation has been completed, as indicated in Fig. 1. Acutely ill patients should be stabilized as rapidly as possible and admitted to an intensive care unit for appropriate monitoring and more definitive management. Remember that for acute inhalation of some substances (e.g., smoke, cadmium oxide, NO_2), the onset of manifestations of injury may be delayed, and patients so exposed should be admitted for 24–48 hr or more

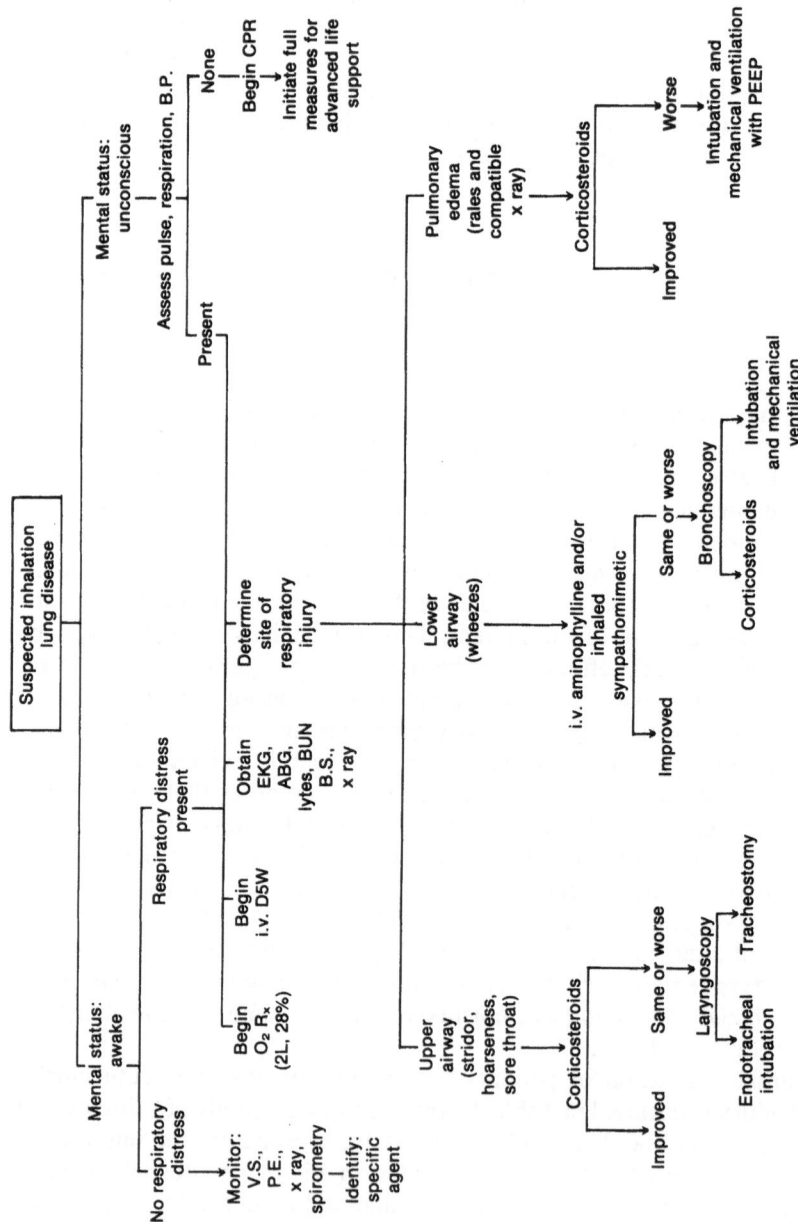

FIGURE 1. Initial management of inhalation lung disease.

TABLE 2. Initial Evaluation of Patients with Known or Possible Acute Inhalational Lung Injury

1. Detailed history of symptoms, circumstances, and nature of exposure, including agent(s) probably involved
2. History of underlying conditions (especially cardiovascular, respiratory, endocrine—e.g. diabetes mellitus)
3. Detailed review of systems
4. Complete physical examination (particular attention to evidence of eye and upper-respiratory injury, skin irritation, dehydration, respiratory rate, rales, rhonchi, wheezes, and other signs of lower-respiratory injury)
5. Complete blood count, basic chemistry (e.g., SMA-18), and urinalysis
6. Arterial blood gas + pH analysis (including carboxyhemoglobin where CO exposure possible)
7. Respiratory flow rates
8. Chest x ray
9. Electrocardiogram
10. Blood and urine for toxicologic analysis where applicable

of observation and monitoring, even if they are in no obvious distress when first seen.

NITROGEN DIOXIDE

Sources of NO_2 exposure are indicated in Table 1. NO_2 is a relatively insoluble gas with a distinctive odor and a yellow–red color, often occurring in combination with other oxides of nitrogen.

The degree of injury caused by NO_2 depends on its concentration and the duration of exposure. The mechanisms of injury include

- Solution in water to form nitric and nitrous acid, nitrites, and nitrates
- Peroxidation of lung lipids and free-radical release
- Formation of methemoglobin
- Degradation of collagen

Because of its low solubility, NO_2 is only mildly irritating to the upper respiratory tract. Consequently, exposed individuals usually inhale the gas for some time without symptoms and contract greater lower-respiratory-tract injury than occurs with more soluble gases. High concentrations of NO_2 may cause acute pulmonary edema (ARDS). Lower concentrations cause injury ranging from alveolar damage (endothelial and epithelial) to bronchial and bronchiolar inflammation and constriction (Table 3).

Occasionally, symptoms occur during exposure to high concentrations; these include transient choking, chest tightness or pain, and profuse

TABLE 3. Clinical Manifestations of NO_2, Cl, and NH_3 Inhalation

Manifestation	NO_2	Cl	NH_3
Relationship of onset to exposure	Latent period, 3–30 hr, then acute onset	Acute onset at time of exposure	Acute onset at time of exposure
External chemical burns on skin	No	No	May be seen
Conjunctival irritation, lacrimation	No	Common	Common and prominent
Nasal irritation, rhinorrhea	No	Common	Common and prominent
Oral and pharyngeal irritation	Uncommon and mild	Common	Common and prominent
Laryngeal edema, stridor, loss of voice	No	May occur	Common
Dyspnea, respiratory distress	Yes	Yes	Yes
Cough, sputum production, hemoptysis	Yes	Yes	Yes; sputum may be copious and watery
Chest pain	Yes; may be pleuritic	Yes; commonly retrosternal	Uncommon
Wheezing, bronchospasm	Common and prominent	May occur	Less common
Rales	Common	May occur	Less common
Pulmonary edema (ARDS)	Common	May occur	Less common
Hypoxemia, cyanosis	Yes	Yes	Yes
Methemoglobinemia	Yes	No	No
Nausea, vomiting	May occur	May occur; may have associated epigastric pain	Less common
Restlessness, anxiety	Yes	Yes	Yes
Fever, tachycardia	Yes	Yes	Yes
Headache	May occur	May occur	May occur
Malaise, weakness	Yes	Yes	Yes
Dehydration, hemoconcentration	Common	May occur	May occur
Leukocytosis, shift to left	Common	May occur	May occur
Systemic hypotension	Common	May occur	May occur
Course	Triphasic—initial acute stage, followed by clinical and radiographic improvement (latent phase—2–6 weeks), followed in some patients by rebound phase; secondary bacterial pneumonia may occur	Rapid recovery with removal from exposure and treatment; secondary bacterial pneumonia may occur	Rapid recovery with removal from exposure and treatment; secondary bacterial (especially *Nocardia*) pneumonia may occur

TABLE 4. Nitrogen Dioxide Inhalation—Clinical Course

	Duration	Clinical features	Chest x ray
Acute phase	3–7 days	Pulmonary edema/ ARDS, bronchitis/ bronchiolitis, broncho- spasm, methemoglobi- nemia, refractory hy- poxemia	Pulmonary edema
Latent phase	2–6 weeks	Slow resolution of fea- tures present in acute phase	Resolving pulmonary edema
Third phase	Weeks–months	Fever, progressive dys- pnea, respiratory in- sufficiency, bronchio- litis obliterans	Nodular interstitial pattern or pulmo- nary edema (occa- sionally)

sweating. Typically, however, there is a latent period of 3–30 hr before the abrupt onset of symptoms.

The clinical course following NO_2 inhalation disease is summarized in Table 4. Not all survivors of the first two phases develop the third. Some survivors of the third phase continue to have residual pulmonary dysfunction. The clinical presentation in phases 1 and 3 may be easily mistaken for acute myocardial infarction or acute infectious pneumonia. It is important to recognize the pattern of this illness (Tables 3 and 4) and the setting in which it occurs (Table 1) in order to make the correct diagnosis and direct therapy.

In the agricultural setting, NO_2 toxicity or silo-filler's disease occurs in conjunction with silo filling in the fall of the year. It must be distinguished from farmer's lung or hypersensitivity pneumonitis, which is more prevalent in winter and spring and is caused by inhalation of spores from moldy hay. In farmer's lung, injury results from a hypersensitivity reaction, not chemical injury.

All patients with suspected NO_2 inhalation should be hospitalized for a 48- to 72-hr period of observation because of the delayed onset of symptoms following exposure. Those who recover from the acute phase need close observation for 6–8 weeks to allow early diagnosis and treatment of the third phase.

Treatment of the acute phase of NO_2 toxicity includes measures directed toward maintenance of adequate gas exchange (see ARDS in Chapter 6) and relief of bronchospasm (see Chapter 11, Asthma). In addition, corticosteroids are helpful (dosage: 40–80 mg prednisone daily) and should probably be maintained for 8 weeks to abort the third phase and prevent bronchiolitis obliterans. Patients not taking corticosteroids should begin them at the first signs of the third phase. Methylene blue (dosage: 2 mg/kg i.v.) may be helpful in the acute phase for reversal of proven methemoglobinemia when oxygenation is seriously impaired, although its use is controversial. There is no proven efficacy for either prophylactic antibiotics or hyperbaric oxygen, which may have adverse effects.

CHLORINE

Chlorine is a greenish-yellow gas with a specific gravity about 2.5 times that of air. In contrast to NO_2, chlorine is highly soluble in water and may cause significant injury to the mucous membranes of the eyes and upper respiratory tract (Tables 1 and 3). Chlorine reacts with water, resulting in the production of hydrochloric acid, hypochlorous acid, and unstable oxidizing agents. This combination of chemicals may lead to more tissue damage than would be produced by equivalent amounts of hydrochloric acid alone.

The effects of chlorine gas are dependent on the dose and duration of exposure. Exposure to 3–5 parts per million (ppm) for brief periods of time may be tolerated without significant injury; 5–8 ppm for a sufficient period of time may cause mild acute illness; 14–21 ppm causes significant injury; and ARDS occurs with exposure to levels greater than 40 ppm (Tables 1 and 3). The effects of exposure are also intensified by the presence of pre-existing disease, especially respiratory or cardiovascular conditions, and the very young and the aged are more severely affected. Common sources of exposure to chlorine gas are listed in Table 1.

Clinical manifestations of chlorine gas inhalation are indicated in Table 3. Symptoms usually have their onset at the time of exposure. These symptoms may be quite marked, but rapid recovery usually occurs upon removal of the patient from the area of contamination. With exposure to higher concentrations, obvious clinical pulmonary edema (i.e., ARDS) with frothy, pink sputum may be noted. In these cases, the chest x ray shows a bilateral acinar-filling pattern that is radiographically indistinguishable from other forms of noncardiogenic pulmonary edema. In some cases, clearing of the pulmonary edema over a few days may be followed by development of bronchopneumonic consolidation, probably due to secondary infection. In cases of severe exposure, arterial hypoxemia, chest x-ray changes, and symptoms may persist at a severe level for 48 hr or more, and complete resolution of symptoms may take several weeks, even with appropriate therapy. Occasionally, the onset of pulmonary edema may be delayed for up to 48 hr after exposure.

Treatment depends on the degree of exposure and the extent of upper- and lower-respiratory findings. All patients should be removed from the area of exposure and put at bed rest. Arterial blood gas (ABG) analysis is mandatory, and most patients will require supplemental oxygen. Severe nasopharyngeal and/or laryngeal edema may require endotracheal intubation or tracheostomy. Severe cases with ARDS should be treated appropriately (see Chapter 6). The role of corticosteroids is uncertain but their use has been recommended by some. Antibiotics should be reserved for actual infection and should not be used prophylactically.

AMMONIA

Ammonia (NH_3) is highly water soluble and exposure causes chemical injury predominantly to the eyes, skin, and upper respiratory tract (Tables 1 and 3). Lower-respiratory-tract involvement is seen less often, but changes indistinguishable from those seen with chlorine have been reported with exposure to very high concentrations of NH_3. Common sources of NH_3 exposure are listed in Table 1.

Symptoms occur coincident with exposure and are indicated in Table 3. With exposure to very high concentrations, severe laryngeal edema may occur and may be fatal. In occasional patients exposed to very high concentrations, ARDS may occur. In patients who survive the initial injury, complicating secondary pulmonary infection by bacteria or *Nocardia asteroides* may develop.

There is poor correlation between severity of clinical disease and chest roentgenographic appearance; the chest x ray may be normal or show evidence of pulmonary edema.

Clinical signs may be the best guide to prognosis in NH_3 inhalation. Patients with no abnormal physical signs in the chest generally recover within 24 hr, whereas those with clinical evidence of pulmonary involvement usually have a more protracted and complicated course, including the development of secondary pulmonary infection. The majority of patients who survive the acute injury recover completely, albeit slowly, but occasional patients have been reported to have residual bronchiectasis and obliteration of small airways.

Severely affected individuals may require aggressive therapy. Laryngeal edema with stridor and loss of voice requires immediate endotracheal intubation or tracheostomy; ARDS should be treated as outlined in Chapter 6. The role of corticosteroid therapy is controversial. In view of the risk of development of significant secondary pulmonary infection, caution should be exercised in administering steroids. The development of infection requires the administration of appropriate antibiotics. There is no evidence that prophylactic antibiotics have any role, and their use may result in the selection of resistant organisms.

SMOKE INHALATION AND CARBON MONOXIDE POISONING

Direct thermal burns of the lower respiratory tract are rare. Except in cases of inhalation of steam where injury to the entire tracheobronchial tree may occur, the inhalation of hot air usually causes injury only as far down as the upper trachea. The upper airway cools inhaled hot air and protects the lower respiratory tract from thermal damage. Therefore, the primary cause of lung injury in victims of fires is from inhalation of toxic gases and particulate matter, rather than thermal injury.

The nature and degree of injury caused by smoke inhalation vary with the constituents of the smoke and the conditions of exposure. Common toxic constituents of smoke are listed in Table 5.

Severe respiratory injury, tissue hypoxia, and lactic acidosis may occur in the absence of cutaneous or respiratory tract burns. The following factors are responsible:

- Ambient oxygen concentration in the smoke may drop from normal (21%) to as low as 10%
- Carbon monoxide (CO) inhibits oxygen binding to hemoglobin
- Hydrogen cyanide may block cellular oxidative phosphorylation
- Toxic constituents directly injure (nitrogen and sulfur oxides) the airways and alveolar–capillary units and inhibit normal metabolism and repair (aldehydes) causing inflammation, wheezing or stridor, and capillary leak
- When present, distant cutaneous thermal burns release endogenous substances that injure pulmonary capillary endothelium (e.g., microemboli, disseminated intravascular coagulation), causing capillary leak

The early manifestations of respiratory injury from smoke inhalation occur within minutes to hours of exposure. They are summarized in Table 6. Although acute obstructive laryngeal edema is rare, it must be suspected and treated aggressively (tracheostomy) if present. The specific characteristics of CO intoxication depend on the blood concentration of CO (i.e., % CO–hemoglobin); these are listed separately in Table 7. The cherry-red color of skin and mucous membranes may help identify patients with high CO levels. Acute myocardial infarction may occur as a complication of tissue hypoxia in this acute phase.

Following the acute phase, some patients with cough and sore throat may clear rapidly, only to relapse within 8–24 hr with recurrent cough, hoarseness, tenacious sputum, and chest pain.

The two most common late complications following smoke inhalation are pulmonary edema and bacterial pneumonia. Pulmonary edema occurs

TABLE 5. Toxic Inhalants Commonly Produced in Fires

Carbon monoxide	Toluene diisocyanate
Nitrogen oxides	Hydrogen cyanide
Hydrogen chloride gas	Sulfur oxides
Aldehydes	Particulates

TABLE 6. Clinical Features of Smoke Inhalation

I. Early manifestations
  A. Subjective
      Sore throat
      Hoarseness
      Cough (dry or productive)
      History of sputum production (thick, tenacious, sooty material)
      Choking sensation
      Dyspnea
      Chest pain
      Headache
      CNS symptoms
      History of loss of consciousness
  B. Objective
    1. Physical examination
      Singed hair on face or in nose
      Singed nosetip
      Burns around lips
      Inflamed oropharyngeal mucosa
      Evidence of surface burns, especially on face
      Respiratory distress
      Inspiratory stridor
      Rarely, acute upper-airway obstruction
      Rales, rhonchi
      Cough productive of sooty material
      Abnormal vital signs
      Cherry-pink color of skin and/or mucous membranes
      Cyanosis
      Confusion, disorientation, somnolence
      Mental obtundation
      Loss of consciousness
      Neurologic findings
    2. Laboratory findings
      Chest x ray usually normal
      Spirometry—reduced respiratory flow rates may be present
      Lung volumes—restrictive ventilatory impairment may be present
      ABGs—hypoxemia may be present
            PCO_2 nl, ↑ or ↓
            pH nl, ↑, ↓
      Carboxyhemoglobin saturation ↑ (>10%)
      Sputum gram stain and culture usually normal
      EKG variable
      CBC variable
II. Later manifestations and complications
  A. Pulmonary edema may be due to:
    1. ARDS
    2. Left ventricular failure
    3. Overzealous fluid administration
  B. Bacterial pneumonia
    1. Frequently gram-negative microorganisms
  C. Bronchiolitis obliterans
    1. Rare
III. Risk factors for complications
  A. Background of smoking
  B. Background of respiratory disease
  C. Background of cardiovascular disease

TABLE 7. Clinical Features of Carbon Monoxide
Intoxication

Level of CO–Hgb	Clinical manifestation
10–20%	Mild headache
	Occasionally mild dyspnea
20–30%	Throbbing headache
	Weakness
	Giddiness on exertion
30–40%	Irritability
	Nausea
	Dizziness
	Dimness of vision
40–50%	Potentially life-threatening
	Confusion
	Ataxia
	Tachypnea
	Tachycardia
50–60%	Commonly fatal
	Stupor
	Convulsions
	Collapse
70–80%	Coma
	Cardiorespiratory depression
>80%	Death virtual certainty

within hours to days of exposure and may be due to toxic injury to the alveolar–capillary membrane (ARDS) or iatrogenic fluid overload. Often, measurement of the pulmonary capillary wedge pressure (by Swan–Ganz catheter) is required to distinguish these two mechanisms.

Smoke inhalation impairs alveolar macrophage function and chemotaxis; this may contribute to the incidence of bacterial pneumonia, which occurs several weeks after the exposure. Clinical features are not different from those of other bacterial pneumonias (see Chapter 4), except that gram-negative organisms are predominant pathogens.

Bronchiolitis obliterans is a rare late complication of smoke inhalation, developing weeks to months after exposure.

All patients with suspected smoke inhalation should be admitted to the hospital to be monitored for 48 hr, because the onset of symptoms may be delayed. Periodic monitoring of asymptomatic patients should include: vital signs, physical examination, chest x ray, and spirometry. If any of these factors deteriorates, ABGs should be obtained. CO levels should be measured. Normal initial spirometry in patients without dermal injury makes later deterioration less likely.

The treatment of smoke inhalation depends in part on the manifestations present in the individual (Table 8). For lower-airway obstruction (wheezes) bronchoscopy may help assess the severity of injury, and bronchodilators should be given (see Chapter 11 for dosage). For upper-airway obstruction (stridor), laryngoscopy may be helpful, and when necessary, endotracheal intubation (by an experienced practitioner) is preferred to maintain an open airway. Occasionally, tracheostomy may be needed. The administration of 100% humidified oxygen (nonrebreathing mask with an oxygen reservoir) will hasten the elimination of high levels of CO. Measurements of CO saturation over 30% must be repeated every 30–60 min. Note that although the ABG measurement of Pa_{O_2} may be only modestly reduced or normal, the blood's oxygen content is reduced by the percentage of measured CO. The patient with CO saturation greater than 30% runs a high risk for hypoxic complications such as myocardial infarction.

When pulmonary edema occurs and is established to be noncardiogenic (by finding a normal pulmonary capillary wedge pressure), it should be treated as outlined in Chapter 6.

Both corticosteroid and prophylactic antibiotic therapy are controversial in the treatment of smoke inhalation. Corticosteroids may be given to patients with airway obstruction (upper or lower) or pulmonary edema for a short period of 24–48 hr. Recommended doses range from 100 mg hydrocortisone every 6 hr for bronchospasm to 30 mg/kg of body weight methylprednisolone every 6–8 hr for ARDS.

Whether or not prophylactic antibiotics are used, it is very important to periodically examine the patient's sputum (smear and culture) for the emergence of significant pathogens, which may need to be treated if clinical signs of infectious bronchitis or pneumonitis develop.

TABLE 8. Management of Smoke Inhalation

Emergency on-the-scene treatment
  Remove victim from scene
  Establish airway if indicated
  Administer supplemental O_2
Treatment of carbon monoxide intoxication
  High concentration (preferably 100%) oxygen
Treatment of lower-airway obstruction
  Oxygen
  Humidify airway with aerosolized water
  Bronchodilators
Treatment of upper-airway obstruction
  Humidify airway
  Severe laryngeal edema dictates endotracheal intubation or tracheostomy
  Corticosteroids
Management of pulmonary edema (see Chapter 6)

OTHER NONMETALLIC GASES

Acetaldehyde

Acetaldehyde (Table 1) has both highly irritant and narcotic properties. Exposure to low concentrations results in eye and upper-respiratory irritation, and exposure to high concentrations may lead to headache, stupor, and ARDS. In the case of the latter, there may be a latent period of 24–48 hr before it becomes manifest. When patients have been exposed to high concentrations of acetaldehyde, they should be observed closely for at least 48 hr because of a possible delay in the development of pulmonary edema.

Acrolein

Acrolein (Table 1) usually exists in a liquid state, but its high vapor pressure may lead to the production of a gas. The intensely irritating effects of this gas on the eyes and upper respiratory tract are impossible to tolerate for more than a brief period of time. Thus, lower-respiratory injury is averted in most cases. Occasionally, inhaling high concentrations of the gas may result in ARDS. The treatment of this complication is as outlined in Chapter 6. Lower-respiratory-tract injury due to acrolein may result in permanent lung damage.

Hydrogen Chloride

Hydrogen chloride (HCl) (Table 1) is the vapor form of hydrochloric acid. This gas is highly irritating to the upper respiratory tract, and exposed individuals often escape the contaminated area before there has been sufficient exposure for lower-respiratory-tract injury to occur. In some circumstances (e.g., fires), however, significant concentrations of HCl may be inhaled resulting in, not only upper-respiratory-tract irritation including glottal edema, but also acute bronchitis and ARDS. When these occur, the treatment is the same as for other irritant gases causing such effects.

Hydrogen Fluoride

Hydrogen fluoride (Table 1) is highly irritating to the skin and mucous membranes, and exposure results in burning of the nose, mouth, and throat, as well as the development of ARDS and pneumonia. The latter two conditions often have their onset after a latent period of 12–24 hr. Management of these complications is as outlined in Chapters 4 and 6. Corticosteroids are generally recommended.

Hydrogen Sulfide

Hydrogen sulfide (Table 1) has both irritant and central nervous system respiratory depressant properties. Exposure to very high concentrations (greater than 700 ppm) results in death from central respiratory depression before there is an opportunity for irritant effects to occur. Exposure to lower levels for prolonged periods of time can result in irritation of both the upper and lower respiratory tracts, with the development of ARDS. Treatment of central respiratory depression requires mechanically assisted ventilation, while ARDS should be managed as outlined in Chapter 6.

Phosgene

Phosgene (carbonyl chloride) (Table 1) is relatively insoluble and, therefore, has little effect on the eyes or upper respiratory tract. Thus, significant quantities of the gas are inhaled without symptoms, causing injury to the lower respiratory tract. ARDS may develop after a latent period of 24–48 hr. Management is as outlined in Chapter 6.

Phosphine

Phosphine (hydrogen phosphide) (Table 1) has a foul, offensive smell that generally limits exposure. With sufficient exposure, however, ARDS may develop, usually after a latent period of 24 hr to several days. Treatment is as outlined in Chapter 6. Owing to the relatively long latent period for the development of pulmonary edema, exposed individuals who appear asymptomatic must be kept under close observation for at least 1 week.

Sulfur Dioxide

Sulfur dioxide (Table 1) is said to be the most commonly encountered toxic gas. When in contact with mucosal surfaces, it is hydrated and oxidized to sulfuric acid and causes severe respiratory tract irritation. The degree of toxicity varies with the level of exposure, ranging from minimal irritation of the upper and/or lower respiratory tract to marked ARDS. High-level exposure may result in severe damage to the upper respiratory tract with severe upper respiratory obstruction. Treatment includes management of ARDS when this develops (Chapter 6) and intubation for upper respiratory obstruction.

INHALATION OF METALS AND METAL COMPOUNDS

Metal Fume Fever

Metal fume fever occurs as a result of exposure to a variety of metal fumes (Table 1). The clinical manifestations are listed in Table 9. Symptoms usually have their onset a few hours after exposure. Although troublesome, the disease is benign and self-limited, with complete resolution usually occurring within 24 hr of removal from exposure. Repeated exposure commonly results in the development of tolerance; this tolerance is lost on cessation of exposure. Treatment is symptomatic.

Cadmium Oxide

Cadmium oxide fumes may cause an acute illness that is initially indistinguishable from metal fume fever, but which may have more significant consequences. Exposure to toxic concentrations of cadmium oxide occurs primarily in occupational settings (Table 1). The effects of cadmium oxide fume exposure are delayed, and there are usually no symptoms during the period of exposure. Cadmium oxide is highly soluble in body fluids and is readily absorbed into the blood following inhalation. It may cause respiratory tract injury including tracheobronchial inflammation and ARDS, as well as nephrotoxicity and hepatotoxicity. Clinical manifestations are listed in Table 9. The onset of symptoms is similar to that of metal fume fever. In addition, there may be associated abdominal cramps and diarrhea. Often the initial improvement resembles the course of metal fume fever, but it is followed in 12–36 hr by the onset of ARDS. Nephrotoxicity may be indicated by the presence of proteinuria, while hepatotoxicity may be suggested by increased liver enzyme and bilirubin levels. The chest x ray reveals evidence of pulmonary edema, which may take from a week to several months to resolve. Death may occur owing to respiratory or renal failure. Cadmium oxide toxicity may be distin-

TABLE 9. Clinical Manifestations of Metal Fume Fever, Cadmium Oxide Fume Fever, and Polymer Fume Fever

Manifestations	Metal fume fever	Cadmium oxide fume fever	Polymer fume fever
Latent period between exposure and onset	2–4 hr	2–4 hr	2–4 hr
Initial phase			
Thirst	Yes	Yes	Yes
Dry throat	Yes	Yes	Yes
Nonproductive cough	Yes	Yes	Yes
Fever	Yes	Yes	Yes
Shaking chills	Yes	Yes	Yes
Diaphoresis	Yes	Yes	Yes
Malaise	Yes	Yes	Yes
Fatigue	Yes	Yes	Yes
Myalgia	Yes	Yes	Yes
Arthralgias	Yes	Yes	Yes
Aching chest discomfort	Yes	Yes	Yes
Dyspnea	Yes	Yes	Yes
Nausea	Yes	Yes	Yes
Headache	Yes	Yes	Yes
Tachycardia	Yes	Yes	Yes
Scattered pulmonary rales	Occasional	Occasional	Occasional
Chest x ray	Usually normal	Usually normal	Usually normal
Polymorphonuclear leukocytosis	Yes	Yes	Yes
Resolution	12–24 hr	12–24 hr but manifestations may persist or recur	24–48 hr
Persistent or recurrent phase	Does not occur	Usually occurs—initial improvement, followed in 12–36 hr by ARDS, hepatotoxicity, and nephrotoxicity	Does not occur
Tolerance on continued exposure	Yes	No	No

guished from metal fume fever by persistent symptoms, especially fever and severe chest pain, beyond 24 hr. Treatment includes warmth and rest, administration of oxygen, ventilatory support, and measures to treat ARDS when this occurs (see Chapter 6). The early use of corticosteroids may improve the prognosis. The use of chelating agents, such as calcium ethylenediamine tetracetic acid, intravenously is controversial; this agent may be nephrotoxic in combination with cadmium.

Mercury Vapor

Exposure to mercury vapor (Table 1) may result in severe tracheo-bronchitis and ARDS. Treatment of toxic inhalation of mercury vapor includes oxygen, other appropriate support, such as aerosol treatment, bronchodilators, and hydration, and corticosteroids.

Other Metals

Other metals and metal compounds that may cause acute respiratory injury (including ARDS) are nickel carbonyl, selenium compounds, titanium tetrachloride, vanadium, and zirconium (Table 1).

POLYMER FUME FEVER

Polymer fume fever is a generally benign, self-limited disorder that is seen in individuals exposed to pyrolysis products of polytetrafluoroethylene resin (Teflon). Such exposure occurs in a variety of occupational and other settings. Individuals using the material may be exposed upon smoking cigarettes that have become contaminated.

Symptoms generally develop after a latent period of 3–4 hr following the onset of exposure (Table 9). Physical examination of the chest is usually unremarkable, although scattered rales may be heard occasionally. The chest x ray is usually normal. The condition is self-limited, and complete recovery generally occurs within 1–2 days, with only symptomatic therapy being needed. In rare cases, ARDS has been reported. The disorder is similar in many respects to metal fume fever, except that tolerance does not develop with repeated exposure.

PARAQUAT POISONING

Although paraquat poisoning is not an inhalational respiratory disease, it merits consideration because of the profound effects that it may have on the lungs. Paraquat is an herbicide that may cause serious and often fatal pulmonary disease when ingested or absorbed through the skin. It does not cause a significant problem when inhaled, probably owing to the upper respiratory tract's elimination of the large particles. The clinical manifestations of paraquat poisoning depend on the dose and route of exposure (Table 10).

TABLE 10. Clinical Manifestations of Paraquat Poisoning

Oral ingestion and gastrointestinal absorption—high dose
  Vomiting, abdominal pain, diarrhea
  Burning, redness, and ulceration of mouth and pharynx
  Severe, rapidly progressive ARDS
Oral ingestion and gastrointestinal absorption—lower dose
  More protracted ARDS
  Renal and hepatic dysfunction
Percutaneous absorption
  Less severe disease
  No oral, pharyngeal, or gastrointestinal problems
  May have reddening, burning, and ulceration of skin at site of absorption

Paraquat generates superoxide radicals, which may be important in the pathogenesis of its effects. Because of this, and in spite of the severe, refractory hypoxemia that is usually encountered, oxygen therapy may be contraindicated, as oxygen may increase the production and/or enhance the toxic effects of superoxide. For this reason, administration of the enzyme superoxide dismutase intravenously or by nebulized aerosol has been suggested for therapy. The use of high doses of corticosteroids is also recommended.

INSECTICIDES

Organophosphates (e.g., parathion, malathion) may cause pulmonary edema and ARDS. More typically, however, when absorbed through the skin, gastrointestinal tract, or lungs, these agents cause systemic toxicity by inhibiting the enzyme acetylcholinesterase, hence producing excessive cholinergic activity. Specific effects include nausea, vomiting, diarrhea, involuntary defecation and urination, blurring of vision, miosis, sweating, lacrimation, salivation, muscle twitching, fasciculations, weakness, flaccid paralysis, cardiac arrhythmias, seizures, electroencephalogram abnormalities, coma, and respiratory depression. Treatment includes atropine, respiratory support, and other measures as indicated.

HYDROCARBON INJURY

Volatile fluorocarbons and chlorinated hydrocarbons (Table 1), when inhaled in sufficient concentration, diffuse across the alveolar capillary membrane into the bloodstream. Their primary toxicity is extrapulmonary rather than pulmonary; they mainly injure the heart, causing conduction defects and cardiac arrhythmias. There is an increased sensitization of the myocardium to sympathomimetic amines, which is intensified by hypoxemia, hypercapnia, stress, and physical activity. These agents also have central nervous system effects, including euphoria, hallucinations, and central nervous system depression. Pulmonary complications, including infection, aspiration, central hypoventilation, and ARDS, are secondary to the cardiac and central nervous system dysfunction. Inhalation may also produce renal and hepatocellular damage. Treatment should be administered in an intensive care unit where appropriate monitoring, supportive therapy, and expectant management of these complications can be accomplished.

Accidental or intentional ingestion of liquid hydrocarbons (kerosene, furniture polish, lighter fluid, paint thinner, gasoline, dry cleaning fluid, insecticides, and other household materials), especially by children, is a common cause of acute pulmonary injury, probably due to vomiting and the aspiration of the hydrocarbon-containing gastric contents into the lung.

Clinically, patients present with burning and evidence of irritation of the mouth and pharynx; there is rapid development of dyspnea, cyanosis, tachypnea, tachycardia, and wheezing. Chest x ray taken with 1–12 hr following ingestion shows patchy air space consolidation and alveolar infiltrates in the dependent portions of the lungs, which may progress to diffuse pulmonary edema and full-blown ARDS. ABG analysis usually reveals hypoxemia and hypocapnia. Since these agents may depress the central nervous system, respiratory depression and carbon dioxide retention may be present. The diagnosis may be suspected from the odor of the ingested agent on the victim's breath. Management of ARDS is reviewed in Chapter 6. Therapy for acute aspiration of gastric contents is reviewed in Chapter 4. Gastric lavage should never be attempted without first inserting a cuffed endotracheal tube to protect the airway and lungs from further aspiration of this material.

ACUTE SILICOSIS

This is a rare condition that occurs as a consequence of exposure in a confined space to very high concentrations of quartz, cristobalite, or tridymite dust of very small particle size. It has been described to occur in association with tunneling through rock of high quartz content, shoveling, loading, and otherwise handling rock dusts in the holds of ships, sand blasting with quartzite sands, and in abrasive soap factories. It is exclusively an occupational disease.

Symptoms usually have their onset within a few weeks of exposure

TABLE 11. Clinical Manifestations of Acute Silicosis

Onset relatively sudden, usually within a few weeks of exposure
Rapidly progressive dyspnea
Malaise, fatigue, weight loss
Cough productive of mucoid sputum, hemoptysis
Pleuritic chest pain
Dyspnea at rest, orthopnea
Central cyanosis
Fever (up to 40°C)
Clubbing
Pleural friction rub
Altered percussion note
Diminished/bronchial breath sounds
Crepitant rales
Severe restrictive ventilatory impairment
Decreased diffusing capacity
Arterial hypoxemia
Chest roentgenogram:
   Diffuse haziness in lower lung fields
   Ground-glass appearance of all lung fields
   Alveolar-filling, pulmonary edema pattern
   Miliary pattern, predominantly lower lung, in some cases
   Diffuse pleural thickening in a few cases

but may, on occasion, take a year or 2 to develop. The predominant complaint is generally rapidly progressive shortness of breath, usually of sudden onset. Other symptoms and clinical manifestations are listed in Table 11. In some cases, the physical examination may be entirely normal.

Sputum examination often reveals strongly PAS-positive material, and electron microscopy of sputum may disclose the presence of lamellar inclusion bodies.

The diagnosis depends on obtaining an accurate exposure history. Individuals who develop acute silicosis usually do not have established chronic silicosis. The differential diagnosis includes pulmonary edema of varying types, idiopathic interstitial fibrosis, sarcoidosis, tuberculosis, various pneumonias, and idiopathic alveolar proteinosis.

The prognosis of this condition is extremely poor, and the majority of patients die within 1 year of the onset of symptoms as a result of cardiorespiratory failure. Those patients who do not die so acutely often have severe residual pulmonary fibrosis.

Corticosteroids are without benefit in this condition. Methods of treatment found successful in idiopathic alveolar proteinosis may be of benefit in acute silicosis, including bronchopulmonary lavage with isotonic saline and inhalation of a trypsin aerosol, but this remains to be established. Infections with mycobacteria and fungi are common complications; patients should be monitored for these and appropriately treated when necessary.

BIBLIOGRAPHY

1. Beach FXM, Jones ES, Scarrow GD: Respiratory effects of chlorine gas. *Br J Indust Med* 26:231, 1969.
2. Bledsoe FH, Seymour EQ: Acute pulmonary edema associated with parathion poisoning. *Radiology* 103:53, 1972.
3. Chester EH, Kaimal J: Pulmonary injury following exposure to chlorine gas: possible beneficial effects of steroid treatment. *Chest* 72:247, 1977.
4. Clutton-Brock J: Two cases of poisoning by contamination of nitrous oxide with higher oxides of nitrogen during anesthesia. *Br J Anaesth* 39:338, 1967.
5. Connolly ME: Paraquat poisoning. *Proc Roy Soc Med* 68:441, 1975.
6. Davis DS, Connolly ME: Paraquat poisoning: Possible therapeutic approach. *Proc Roy Soc Med* 68:442, 1975.
7. Eade NR, Taussig LM, Marks MI: Hydrocarbon pneumonitis. *Pediatrics* 54:351, 1974.
8. Epstein PE: Aspiration disease of the lungs, in Fishman AP (ed): *Pulmonary Diseases and Disorders*. New York, McGraw-Hill, 1980, pp 1327.
9. Horvath EP, doPuio GA, Barbee RA, Dicke HA: Nitrogen dioxide-induced pulmonary disease. *J Occup Med* 20:103, 1978.
10. Kurtz WD, McCord CP: Polymer-fume fever. *J Occup Med* 16:480, 1974.
11. Lakshminarayan S: Inhalation injury of the lungs, in Sahn SA (ed): *Pulmonary Emergencies*. New York, Churchill Livingstone, 1982, p 375.
12. Larkin JM, Brokos GJ, Moylon JA: Treatment of carbon monoxide poisoning: Prognostic factors. *J Trauma* 16:111, 1976.
13. McArdle CS, Finlay WF: Pulmonary complications following smoke inhalation. *Br J Anaesth* 47:618, 1978.
14. Montague TJ, MacNeil AR: Mass ammonia inhalation. *Chest* 77:496, 1980.
15. Parks WR: *Occupational Lung Disorders*, ed 2. London, Butterworths, 1982, p 454.
16. Sobonya R: Fatal anhydrous ammonia inhalation. *Hum Pathol* 8:293, 1977.
17. Xipell JM, Ham KN, Price CG, Thomas DP: Acute silicoproteinosis. *Thorax* 32:104, 1977.
18. Yockey CC, Eden BM, Byrd RB: The McConnell missle accident: Clinical spectrum of nitrogen dioxide exposure. *JAMA* 244:1221, 1981.

CHAPTER 6

Pulmonary Edema

Philip Witorsch and Ann Medinger

INTRODUCTION

Definition

Pulmonary edema is a pathologic state in which there is an excessive accumulation of fluid in the extravascular tissues of the lung. It occurs when the balance of factors governing movement of fluid across the alveolar–capillary membrane (hydrostatic and osmotic pressure gradients and the permeability characteristics of the capillary wall, described in Fig. 1) shifts to allow more fluid to be filtered from the pulmonary capillaries than can be removed by vascular reabsorption and lymphatic clearance.

Physiologic Classification

Pulmonary edema is classified according to the permeability characteristics of the alveolar–capillary membrane (Table 1). In increased permeability pulmonary edema (IPPE, high-permeability pulmonary edema, permeability pulmonary edema, primary pulmonary edema, alveolar capillary leak syndrome), there is an increase in the permeability

Philip Witorsch • Respiratory Care, Division of Pulmonary Diseases and Allergy, George Washington University School of Medicine and Health Sciences, Washington, D.C., 20037; Georgetown University Schools of Medicine and Dentistry, Washington, D.C. 20007; Center for Environmental Health and Human Toxicology, Washington, D.C., 20007. Ann Medinger • Division of Pulmonary Diseases and Allergy, George Washington University School of Medicine and Health Sciences, Washington, D.C. 20037; Pulmonary Function Laboratory, Veterans Administration Medical Center, Washington, D.C. 20422.

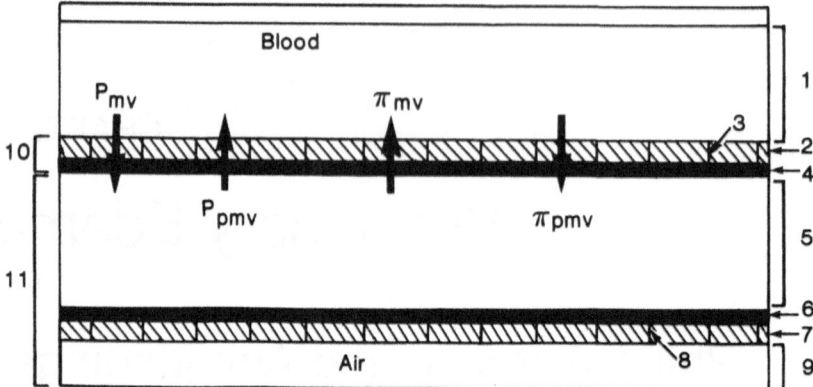

FIGURE 1. Factors governing movement of fluid across the alveolar–capillary "membrane." (1) Alveolar capillary lumen (intravascular space), (2) alveolar-capillary endothelium, (3) endothelial junction, (4) endothelial basement membrane, (5) interstitial space, (6) epithelial basement membrane, (7) alveolar epithelium, (8) alveolar epithelial "tight" junction, (9) alveolar space, (10) alveolar-capillary membrane, (11) extravascular space. Pmv—microvascular (intravascular) hydrostatic pressure, Ppmv—perimicrovascular (interstitial) hydrostatic pressure, πmv—microvascular oncotic (osmotic) pressure, πpmv—perimicrovascular oncotic pressure.

Broad arrows indicate direction of fluid movement resulting from increase in that factor. Fluid movement from intravascular to extravascular space will be favored by increased Pmv, decreased Ppmv, decreased πmv, increased πpmv, or increased permeability of the alveolar–capillary membrane. The relationship between fluid flow across the alveolar–capillary membrane and these factors is described by the Starling–Landis equation:

$$Q_f = K_f[(Pmv - Ppmv) + \sigma(\pi mv - \pi pmv)]$$

where Q_f = net transvascular flow of fluid, K_f = fluid filtration coefficient, and σ = reflection coefficient (effectiveness of membrane in preventing flow of solute compared to water).

of the alveolar–capillary endothelial membrane, without any primary changes in hydrostatic or oncotic pressure gradients. In normal permeability pulmonary edema (NPPE, hemodynamic pulmonary edema, secondary pulmonary edema), alveolar–capillary endothelial permeability is normal (at least initially) and there is an alteration in the hydrostatic or oncotic pressure gradient. This distinction has practical diagnostic and therapeutic implications.

Examples

A primary change of one type may lead to a secondary change of another type. For example, in neurogenic and high-altitude pulmonary

TABLE 1. Classification, Features, and Treatment of Acute Pulmonary Edema

Physiologic defect and causes	PROT$_{alv}$	Ppa	Ppcw	Specific clinical clues	Specific therapy
I. Increased permeability					
1. ARDS (shock, sepsis, DIC, gastric aspiration, severe pneumonia, etc.—see Table 2)	↑	↑	N[a]	a. Presence of associated conditions/precipitating factors (see Table 2) b. Severe, refractory hypoxemia c. Normal cardiac silhouette on chest x ray[a] d. Decreased compliance	a. Mechanical ventilation b. PEEP c. Oxygen d. Swan–Ganz catheter, precise fluid managment e. ? Corticosteroids f. Treatment of underlying condition(s)
2. Opiates, etc. (opiates, propoxyphene, ethchlorvynol, aspirin, etc.)	↑	N–↑	N	a. History/evidence drug ingestion/administration b. Altered sensorium c. Pupillary abnormalities d. Respiratory depression	a. Mechanical ventilation b. Oxygen c. Naloxone
3. Neurogenic[b] (head trauma, seizures, CVA, etc.)	↑	N–↑	N–↑	a. History of neurologic "event" b. Neurologic findings c. Increased intracranial pressure	a. Oxygen b. Mechanical ventilation c. Specific treatment of underlying neurologic problem
4. High altitude[b]	↑	↑↑	N–↑	a. Occurrence at high altitude b. Acute mountain sickness	a. Oxygen b. Immediate descent to lower altitude

(continued)

TABLE 1. (*continued*)

Physiologic defect and causes	$PROT_{alv}$	Ppa	Ppcw	Specific clinical clues	Specific therapy
II. Normal permeability					
A. ↑ Microvascular hydrostatic P					
1. "Cardiogenic" (aortic valve disease, hypertensive heart disease, ASHD, cardiomyopathy, arrhythmias, constrictive pericarditis, mitral valve disease, left atrial myxoma, etc.)	N	↑	↑ – ↑ ↑	a. Specific cardiac findings on history and physical examination b. Electrocardiographic abnormalities c. Radiographic abnormalities of cardiac silhouette d. Pleural effusion	a. Diuretics b. Morphine c. Oxygen d. Reduction of preload prn e. Reduction of afterload prn
2. Noncardiogenic (high-output states, e.g., thyrotoxicosis, systemic A-V fistula, beriberi, severe anemia, i.v. fluid overload, increased pulm. venous P—e.g., pulm. veno-occlusive disease, fibrosing mediastinitis, congenital vascular abnormalities)	N	↑	↑ – ↑ ↑	a. History, symptoms, physical signs of specific underlying condition b. Radiographic features of specific underlying conditions c. Other laboratory features of specific underlying conditions	a. Treatment of specific underlying condition b. Oxygen c. Diuretics
B. ↓ Perimicrovascular hydrostatic P					

Mechanism				Diagnostic features	Treatment
1. Marked changes in airway and transthoracic pressure (mechanical ventilation at high inspiratory P, high levels of PEEP, upper airway obstruction)	N	N	N N	a. Specific associated circumstances and conditions b. Distinctive physical findings—e.g., inspiratory stridor with upper airway obstruction	a. Correction of specific precipitating factors—e.g., reduction of pressures, relief of upper-airway obstruction b. Oxygen
2. Surfactant depletion (re-expansion of collapsed lung)	N		N	a. Specific associated circumstances and conditions b. Unilateral pulmonary edema	a. Oxygen b. Occasionally, mechanical ventilation
C. ↓ Microvascular osmotic pressure					
1. Severe hypoalbuminemia (usually aggravated by rapid i.v. crystalloid replacement)	N→↓		N	a. Severe hypoalbuminemia b. Recent rapid i.v. crystalloid administration	a. Correct hypoalbuminemia b. Oxygen c. Occasionally, mechanical ventilation
D. ↑ Perimicrovascular osmotic pressure					
1. Lymphatic obstruction (carcinomatosis, lymphangiomyomatosis, pneumoconiosis, prolonged elevation of systemic venous pressure)	N→↑		N	a. Specific associated condition (e.g., carcinomatosis)	a. Oxygen b. Occasionally, mechanical ventilation c. Treatment of underlying condition, if possible (e.g., radiation, chemotherapy)

[a] While Ppcw would be expected to be normal in ARDS uncomplicated by heart failure, in some cases there is associated cardiac decompensation which results in an elevation of the Ppcw and which may also result in an enlarged cardiac silhouette on chest x ray.

[b] While neurogenic and high altitude pulmonary edema are usually classified as increased permeability edema and are associated with elevated $PROT_{alv}$, there is evidence to suggest that in fact the primary initiating mechanism in these conditions may be a hemodynamic one, i.e., pulmonary hypertension with increased hydrostatic pressure, and that the increased permeability that is seen may be a secondary phenomenon.

edema, there is probably an initial marked increase in microvascular hydrostatic pressure; this damages the alveolar–capillary endothelial membrane, resulting in a secondary increase in membrane permeability.

Sometimes, two or more mechanisms of pulmonary edema may be operative simultaneously. For example, a few patients with the adult respiratory distress syndrome (ARDS), which is due to increased capillary permeability, have concurrently increased microvascular hydrostatic pressure, due to left ventricular failure, and/or decreased microvascular oncotic pressure, due to severe hypoproteinemia.

Since ARDS is the most common type of IPPE and cardiac dysfunction is the most common cause of NPPE, most of the subsequent discussion is directed toward diagnosis and management of these two conditions. (See Table 1 for a list of other conditions associated with IPPE and NPPE.)

Neither cardiogenic nor ARDS pulmonary edema is a single disease. *Cardiogenic* pulmonary edema may occur in association with a number of cardiac defects (e.g., coronary artery disease, cardiac valvular dysfunction, myocarditis), all of which cause a rise in hydrostatic pressure within the lung.

ARDS occurs in association with a variety of more diverse diseases or conditions, ranging from trauma to infection (see Table 2), all of which cause a rise in pulmonary–capillary permeability. The list of criteria further defining this syndrome is given in Table 3 and will be discussed further below.

TABLE 2. Conditions Associated with ARDS

Shock (septic, hemorrhagic, cardiogenic, anaphylactic)	Liquid aspiration (gastric juice, fresh and salt water near drowning, hydrocarbons)
Pulmonary infections (viral, fungal, *Pneumocystis carinii,* mycobacterial, *Legionella*, miliary tuberculosis)	Drug overdose (opiates, propoxyphene, ethchlorvynol, barbiturates, paraldehyde, salicylates, etc.)
Nonpulmonary infections (gram-negative sepsis)	Paraquat poisoning
Pancreatitis	Inhaled toxins (nitrogen oxides, chlorine, ammonia, phosgene, cadmium, etc.)
Uremia	High concentrations of oxygen (pulmonary oxygen toxicity)
Lymphangitic carcinomatosis	Massive blood transfusions
Toxemia of pregnancy	Leukocyte transfusions
Postcardioversion	Thoracic trauma
Radiation pneumonitis	Nonthoracic trauma
Acute leukemia	Fat emboli
Air emboli	Some cases of neurogenic pulmonary edema
Amniotic fluid emboli	
Cardiopulmonary bypass	
Smoke inhalation	

TABLE 3. Clinical Features of ARDS

History
  Previously normal lungs
  Presence of an antecedent associated catastrophic medical condition
  Latent period 24–48 hr
  Abrupt onset
Physical examination
  Tachypnea (respirations > 20/min), dyspnea, labored breathing
  Intercostal retractions, use of accessory muscles
  Auscultation
    Normal
    Diffuse rales
    Consolidation
Chest x ray
  Early: normal or interstitial infiltrate
  Later: diffuse alveolar infiltrates (white lung)
  Normal heart size
  No pleural effusion
Pulmonary mechanics
  Reduced compliance (high ventilator cycling pressure)
  Increased dead space
Hemodynamics
  Ppcw < 12 mm Hg Ppa >25 mm Hg
  Normal cardiac output
Arterial blood gas
  Refractory hypoxemia (Pa_{O_2} < 50 mm Hg with $F_{I_{O_2}}$ > 0.6)
  ↓ Pa_{CO_2}, ↓ pH (mixed respiratory alkalosis and metabolic acidosis)
  ↓ $S\bar{v}_{O_2}$, ↑ a-$\bar{v}_{O_2}$ difference
Alveolar fluid/plasma protein ratio
  >0.6

DIFFERENTIAL DIAGNOSIS OF PULMONARY EDEMA

The diagnosis of pulmonary edema requires, first, differentiation of this condition from others that commonly present with acute respiratory distress (pneumonia, pulmonary embolism, airway obstruction). Once the general diagnosis of pulmonary edema is certain, the type of pulmonary edema must be identified and the specific etiology sought (e.g., acute myocardial infarction, toxic exposure) while acute therapeutic measures are begun.

Although *individual* clinical and routine laboratory parameters are usually not definitive in diagnosing pulmonary edema and identifying its etiology, a correct diagnosis can usually be made on the basis of a combination of the findings described below.

History

The history is helpful in differentiating pulmonary edema from other common respiratory emergencies. Pneumonia is usually accompanied by chest pain (often pleuritic), purulent sputum, fever, and chills. Airway diseases usually have an antecedent history of allergy and episodic shortness of breath or chronic progressive dyspnea on exertion with chronic cough and sputum production. Pulmonary embolism usually occurs in patients with predisposing conditions such as recent surgery, recent immobilization during long-distance travel, chronic congestive heart failure, or oral contraceptive usage. It is usually accompanied by chest pain.

Historical information also helps identify the etiology of the pulmonary edema. Features of the history that may help distinguish cardiogenic pulmonary edema from ARDS include: inpatient (ARDS) versus outpatient (cardiogenic) setting; insidious (cardiogenic) versus abrupt (ARDS) onset; history of cardiac symptoms or disease; and history of disease or toxic exposure predisposing the patient to ARDS. These are summarized in Table 4. Clinical characteristics of ARDS are given in Table 3.

Historical clues must be sought to identify pulmonary edema due to opiate and other drug administration, viral pneumonitis, cerebrovascular accident, trauma, gastric aspiration, toxemia of pregnancy, near drowning, or high altitude.

Physical Examination

Patients with pulmonary edema are usually in respiratory distress, with tachypnea, tachycardia, labored respirations, use of accessory muscles of respiration, and often central cyanosis. There is cough, often productive of watery or blood-tinged sputum. Auscultation of the chest may reveal bilateral basilar or diffuse rales, or wheezes and rhonchi. However, in the early stages of pulmonary edema, chest auscultation may be clear.

Several features of the physical examination help distinguish pulmonary edema from respiratory failure due to pneumonia, airway obstruction, and pulmonary embolism. Fever over 38.5°C favors pneumonia; the rales of pneumonia are usually localized and may be accompanied by other signs of local pulmonary consolidation. However, diffuse bilateral bronchopneumonia may sound like pulmonary edema on chest auscultation.

Although patients with chronic airway obstruction may have signs of right-heart failure (jugular venous distention, peripheral edema, and S3 gallop varying with respirations), they also usually have physical signs characteristic of chronic airflow obstruction: barrel-shaped chest, evidence of weight loss, pursed-lip breathing, body positioned leaning for-

TABLE 4. Differential Diagnosis of Cardiogenic Pulmonary Edema versus ARDS

Features favoring cardiogenic pulmonary edema	Features favoring ARDS
Insidious onset	Condition associated with ARDS (see
Outpatient onset	Table 2)
Cardiac history	Abrupt onset
Symptoms of acute MI	Physical signs of consolidation
Blood-tinged or rusty sputum	Clear lungs on auscultation
Frothing, foamy sputum	"White" lung on x ray
Clinical evidence of CHF	Normal cardiac silhouette on x ray
Significant systemic hypertension	Refractory hypoxemia
Rales without consolidation	
EKG evidence of acute MI	
Ischemic ST-T wave changes	
EKG evidence of LVH	
P-wave abnormalities indicative of left atrial enlargement	
Redistribution of pulmonary blood flow to upper zones on x ray	
Cardiomegaly on x ray	
Other x-ray features—see Table 5	
Pleural effusion	
Rapid response to diuretics	

ward braced on outstretched arms, and a hyperresonant chest. Of all the patients with pulmonary edema, those with cardiogenic edema are the most likely to wheeze; these patients can also be recognized by the presence of the additional signs of left-heart dysfunction: S3 gallop rhythm not varying with respirations, enlarged heart, and valvular murmurs.

Patients with pulmonary embolism most often have a normal chest examination; occasionally localized wheezes or a pleural friction rub is heard.

The physical examination is also helpful for identifying the etiology of the pulmonary edema. Wheezing and florid pulmonary edema with rales and foamy, blood-tinged sputum are more often found in cardiogenic pulmonary edema; other signs of cardiac dysfunction have been listed above. In contrast, patients with pulmonary edema due to ARDS often present with minimal auscultatory findings on chest examination in spite of significant respiratory distress. See Table 4 for a summary of clinical factors distinguishing cardiogenic and ARDS pulmonary edema. Clinical characteristics of ARDS are summarized in Table 3.

The physical examination may reveal other evidence of conditions predisposing to ARDS, such as pancreatitis, toxemia of pregnancy, sepsis, or trauma (see Table 2). Needle tracks along peripheral veins suggest opiate-induced pulmonary edema; other signs of opiate use include miosis and hypoventilation. Evidence of head trauma or of central neurologic deficits from cerebral tumor or vascular accident suggests neurogenic pulmonary edema.

Routine Laboratory and X-Ray Studies

The initial laboratory and x-ray studies that are most helpful in diagnosing pulmonary edema and identifying the etiology and severity are

- Chest x ray
- Electrocardiogram (EKG)
- White blood cell count and differential (WBC)
- Arterial blood gases (ABG)

Chest X Ray. In respiratory distress due to airway obstruction or pulmonary embolism, the chest x ray usually reveals an absence of parenchymal infiltrates. In the early stages of pulmonary edema, the chest x ray may also be normal (especially in ARDS) or may show an interstitial pattern; however, it rapidly progresses to the acinar pattern described below.

The chest x ray does not always differentiate pulmonary edema from pneumonia and the less common conditions of alveolar proteinosis, diffuse alveolar cell carcinoma, and interstitial fibrosis. However, in general, if the x ray shows a diffuse bilateral acinar filling pattern, pulmonary edema is likely; if the pattern is acinar, but asymmetric or localized, pneumonia is more likely, though pulmonary edema can also occur in this pattern.

Cardiogenic pulmonary edema has characteristic x-ray features, making it easier to distinguish from other causes of respiratory distress and from other causes of pulmonary edema. These are listed on Table 5. The most helpful and specific x-ray sign of cardiogenic pulmonary edema is vascular redistribution of pulmonary blood flow to the upper lung zones. Cardiomegaly is another helpful sign, but may be absent in cardiogenic pulmonary edema due to acute myocardial infarction, restrictive cardiomyopathy, or left atrial myxoma.

TABLE 5. Cardiogenic Pulmonary Edema: Chest X-Ray Characteristics

Cardiomegaly	Blurring of vascular markings
Aortic valve calcification	Increased bronchial wall thickness
Mitral valve calcification	Air bronchograms
Coronary artery calcification	Silhouette signs
Pleural effusion(s)	Perihilar "butterfly" distribution of
Redistribution of pulmonary blood flow to upper-lung zones (increased caliber of upper-lobe vessels)	infiltrates

Pulmonary edema due to *ARDS* is characterized radiographically by a rapid progression from normal to a diffuse, homogeneous "white" lung, within hours to days. Vascular redistribution is absent; the heart size is usually normal (absent coexisting heart disease) and pleural effusions are usually absent. See Table 3.

EKG. The EKG may disclose evidence of acute or chronic heart disease, which is supportive evidence for cardiogenic pulmonary edema. Look specifically for new Q waves of infarction, ST-T-wave changes of injury and ischemia, and P-wave changes of mitral or left atrial disease. P-wave changes of right atrial disease may help confirm the suspicion that chronic airway obstruction is causing the respiratory distress.

WBC. The WBC helps to distinguish pneumonia from pulmonary edema. Leukocytosis (over 15,000) with a left shift in the differential suggests bacterial pneumonia; this sign is usually absent in viral pneumonia. Remember that bacterial pneumonia may precipitate cardiogenic pulmonary edema in patients with heart disease.

ABG. Although the ABG measurement does not identify patients with pulmonary edema, it does help determine the severity of the gas exchange defect and guide therapy. Hypoxemia is invariably present in pulmonary edema. Severe hypoxemia (Pa_{O_2} < 50 mm Hg on room air) that is refractory to oxygen therapy suggests ARDS, which will probably require intubation and mechanical ventilation. The Pa_{CO_2} is usually reduced, sometimes with an associated respiratory alkalosis, although metabolic (lactic) acidosis may appear as a result of severe hypoxia. Finding an elevated Pa_{CO_2} suggests that there is depression of the respiratory control center (narcotic use), chronic airway obstruction, or such severe respiratory failure that respiratory muscle fatigue has occurred and respiratory arrest may be imminent. When patients with pulmonary edema are found to have a rising Pa_{CO_2} and progressive acidosis, preparations should be promptly made for intubation and mechanical ventilation.

Blood gas and pH measurements can also be made from blood obtained from the main pulmonary artery (through a Swan–Ganz catheter), i.e., mixed venous blood. The measurement of mixed venous oxygen saturation ($S\bar{v}_{O_2}$) gives important information about oxygen uptake and delivery, as will be discussed below.

Clinical Course as a Diagnostic Parameter

Cardiogenic pulmonary edema usually responds rapidly to diuresis and will often resolve within a few hours with such treatment. Most instances of noncardiogenic pulmonary edema, especially ARDS, do not respond to such measures and pursue a course of many hours to many days, even with appropriate therapy. For this reason, a therapeutic–diagnostic trial of furosemide may be helpful in patients with suspected cardiogenic pulmonary edema.

Special Studies

In most patients with pulmonary edema, the more sophisticated diagnostic tests listed below are not necessary for either diagnosis or management.

Hemodynamic Measurements. Hemodynamic measurements are particularly helpful in the following settings:

- Diagnostic: When the nature of the pulmonary edema is unclear.
- Therapeutic: In ARDS, to confirm the diagnosis [normal pulmonary capillary wedge pressure (Ppcw)] and to manage fluid therapy.
- Therapeutic: In cardiogenic pulmonary edema, when there is associated hemodynamic instability.

The hemodynamic measurements that may be made with a Swan–Ganz catheter inserted into the pulmonary artery include pulmonary artery pressures (systolic, diastolic, mean), Ppcw, and cardiac output ($\dot{Q}$). Ppcw is high (above 16 mm Hg) in cardiogenic pulmonary edema and low (below 12 mm Hg) in ARDS, if the measurement is taken before significant diuresis. $\dot{Q}$ is normal in ARDS and low in cardiogenic pulmonary edema. This distinction is lost when mixed defects are present. The hemodynamic characteristics of various types of pulmonary edema are listed in Table 1.

Vital hemodynamic measurements require the use of correct technique in catheter placement, pressure calibration, and measurement. In measuring pressures, extraneous factors such as ventilator pressures must be accounted for.

Edema Fluid Protein Analysis. Measuring edema fluid protein ($Prot_{alv}$) and comparing it to plasma protein ($Prot_{plas}$), clearly distinguishes patients with IPPE, such as ARDS, from those with NPPE, such as cardiogenic pulmonary edema:

	$Prot_{alv}/Prot_{plas}$
IPPE	>0.6
NPPE	<0.6

The techniques for this measurement are not widely available at this time.

TREATMENT

General

The emergency management of pulmonary edema is summarized in Fig. 2. Prior to determining the cause of the pulmonary edema, treatment may be instituted with the following general measures:

- Oxygen: 40–100% mask or 6–8 liters/min nasal prongs
- Furosemide: 20–50 mg i.v. bolus
- Aminophylline: Choose a loading dose and maintenance infusion for patients with heart disease (Chapter 10, Table 2)
- Admit to the intensive care unit: Include bed rest, continuous cardiac monitoring, frequent vital signs, intensive nursing attention

The efficacy of the oxygen therapy must be monitored with serial ABGs to determine the best dose of oxygen with least toxicity, and to avoid the development of CO_2 narcosis in patients with concomitant severe chronic airway obstruction. Never delay the institution of oxygen therapy while awaiting ABG information. Oxygen therapy should *not* be given to patients with possible paraquat-induced pulmonary edema; it may exacerbate the condition.

Diuretic administration is most useful to treat cardiogenic pulmonary edema. Moreover, a single dose is rarely harmful to patients with noncardiogenic pulmonary edema. Clinical improvement after the diuretic may help identify cardiogenic pulmonary edema.

Cardiogenic Pulmonary Edema

When the diagnosis of cardiogenic pulmonary edema is certain, further specific measures may be instituted. These are summarized in Table 6.

Frequently, cardiogenic pulmonary edema can be controlled with supportive care (oxygen, aminophylline, bed rest, morphine, sedation) and preload reduction in the form of diuretic therapy. Further measures that must be undertaken if this treatment is insufficient include afterload reduction, inotropic therapy, and arrhythmia control. Their use depends on identification of the pathophysiologic defect causing the cardiac dysfunction. When they are required, it is often helpful to monitor cardiac hemodynamic measurements (cardiac output, Ppcw, and mean arterial pressure).

The use of digitalis preparations for the treatment of acute cardiogenic pulmonary edema is controversial, because myocardial ischemia is frequently the cause of or a contributor to the left ventricular failure.

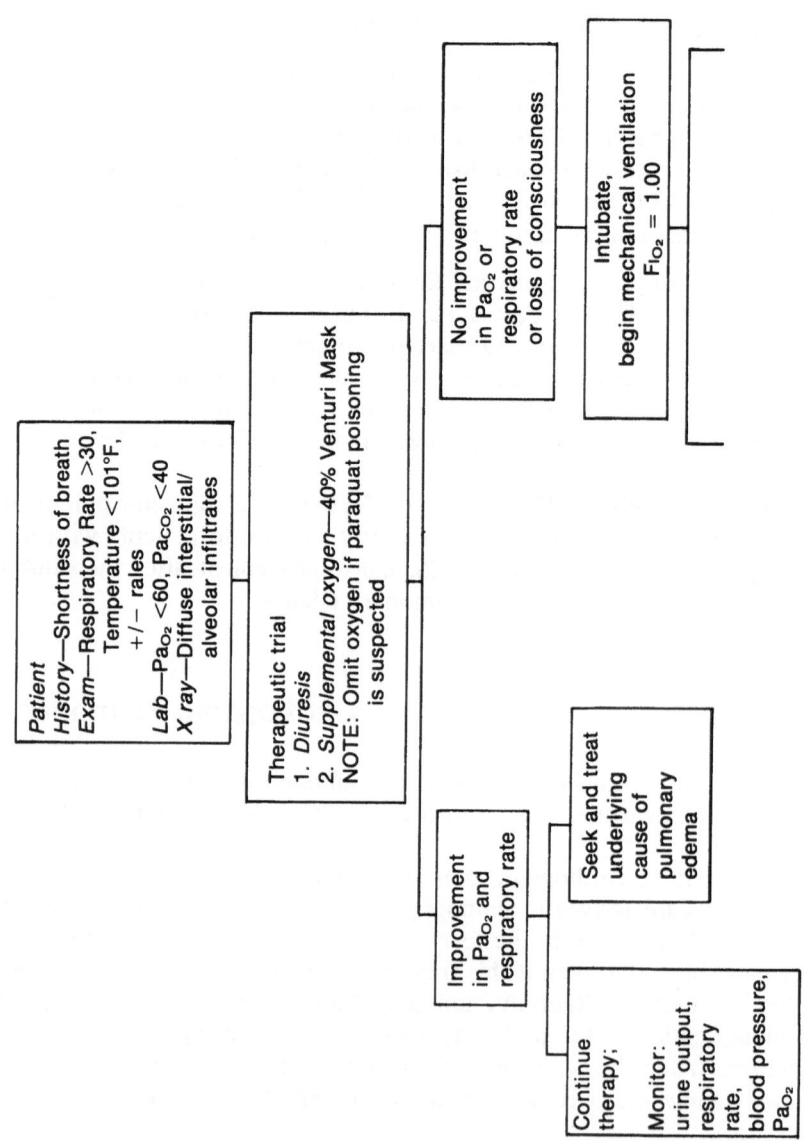

Patient
History—Shortness of breath
Exam—Respiratory Rate >30,
Temperature <101°F,
+/− rales
Lab—Pa_{O_2} <60, Pa_{CO_2} <40
X ray—Diffuse interstitial/
alveolar infiltrates

Therapeutic trial
1. *Diuresis*
2. *Supplemental oxygen*—40% Venturi Mask
NOTE: Omit oxygen if paraquat poisoning
is suspected

Improvement
in Pa_{O_2} and
respiratory rate

No improvement
in Pa_{O_2} or
respiratory rate
or loss of consciousness

Continue
therapy;

Monitor:
urine output,
respiratory
rate,
blood pressure,
Pa_{O_2}

Seek and treat
underlying
cause of
pulmonary
edema

Intubate,
begin mechanical ventilation
$F_{I_{O_2}}$ = 1.00

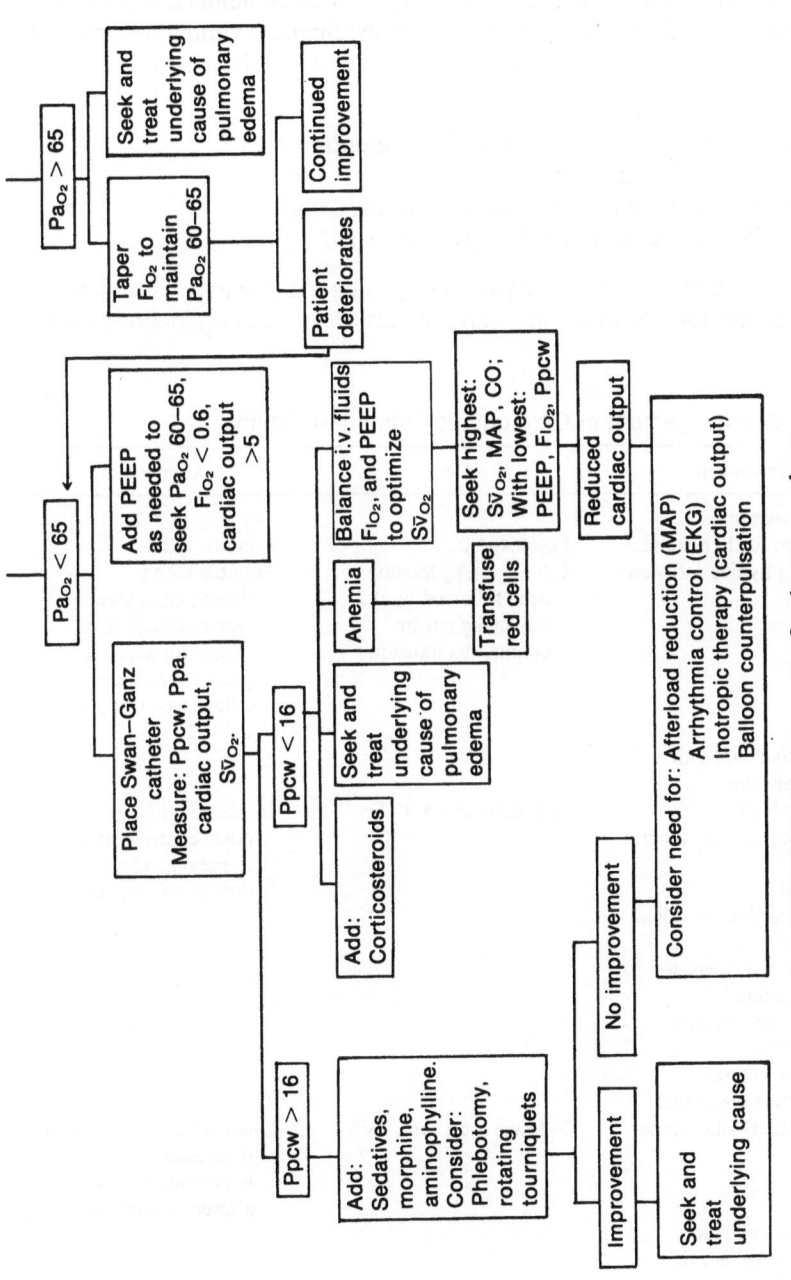

FIGURE 2. Management of pulmonary edema.

Digitalis and most inotropic agents increase myocardial oxygen demand and may exacerbate ischemia. Digitalis toxicity with arrhythmia is also more likely to occur in the presence of myocardial ischemia and hypoxia.

Endotracheal intubation and assisted mechanical ventilation may be required to treat pulmonary edema in the following circumstances:

- Loss of consciousness
- Respiratory depression with CO_2 retention
- Refractory hypoxemia
- Respiratory muscle fatigue with rising Pa_{CO_2}
- Failure to respond to therapy within 1–2 hr

Occasionally, cardiogenic pulmonary edema is due to a massive myocardial infarction with very low cardiac output. In this case balloon coun-

TABLE 6. Management of Cardiogenic Pulmonary Edema

Treatment	Dose	Comments
General measures		
Oxygen for hypoxemia	FI_{O_2} 0.4–1.0	Monitor ABGs
Aminophylline infusion	4.0–5.6 mg/kg loading dose followed by 0.2–0.5 mg/kg per hr continuous infusion	Monitor blood theophylline levels; recommended dose takes into account presence of heart failure, see Chapter 10, Table 2
Intensive care unit monitoring		
Prophylactic subcutaneous heparin	5000 units every 12 hr	In absence of bleeding or other contraindication; to prevent venous thrombosis and emboli
Reduce cardiac workload		
Overall		
Bed rest, bedside commode		
Reduce physical stress		
Stool softener		
Reduce emotional stress—morphine	3–15 mg s.c., i.m., i.v.	Use with extreme caution if alveolar hypoventilation or altered sensoriuom
Preload reduction		
Rotating tourniquets		
Phlebotomy		
Furosemide	20–50 mg i.v., double dose every 2–3 hr until diuresis; do not exceed 240 mg/dose	

TABLE 6. (*continued*)

Treatment	Dose	Comments
Afterload reduction		
Sodium nitroprusside	10–20 μg/min i.v. initially, increments of 5 μg/min every 5 min until pulmonary edema is relieved or systemic arterial systolic BP falls below 100 mm Hg	Arterial cannula for BP monitoring and Swan–Ganz catheter desirable; monitor serum thiocyanate levels
Nitroglycerine	0.3–0.6 mg sublingually	May be hazardous in acute myocardial infarction with normal to reduced BP
Improve myocardial contractility		
Digoxin	0.25–0.5 mg i.v. over several minutes initially in patient known not to be receiving digitalis and with normal renal function; subsequent dosage will depend on clinical course	Use controversial in acute mycardial infarction—may increase myocardial oxygen demand; reduce dosage in renal failure
Dopamine	5–8 μg/kg per min i.v. infusion	In pulmonary edema associated with cardiogenic shock; titrate carefully to avoid precipitating ventricular arrhythmias or severe peripheral vasoconstriction; Swan–Ganz catheter and arterial cannula for BP monitoring desirable
Control arrhythmias		
Supraventricular tachycardia:		
Digoxin	See above	See above
Verapamil	Initial dose of 5–10 mg i.v. over 2–3 min; may be repeated after 30 min p.r.n.	Negative inotropic effects may limit its use in cardiogenic pulmonary edema
Ventricular tachycardia:		
Lidocaine	100-mg i.v. bolus followed in 5 min by 50-mg i.v. bolus; maintenance infusion of 1–4 mg/min	
Cardioversion		
Heart block		
Isoproterenol	i.v. infusion of concentration of 2–4 μg/ml at rate of 2–20 μg/min	Use with extreme caution, if at all, in acute myocardial infarction
Pacemaker		

terpulsation may be required to treat both hypotension and pulmonary edema.

ARDS

In treating ARDS, hospitalization on an intensive care unit, with hemodynamic (i.e., Swan–Ganz), electrocardiographic, and blood gas monitoring, is mandatory. Since there is no specific treatment for ARDS, the overall goals are supportive. The goals of treatment include

- Adequate oxygenation with the least risk of pulmonary oxygen toxicity and barotrauma
- Adequate pulmonary and systemic perfusion with low levels of hydrostatic pressure in the pulmonary vascular bed
- Limiting further pulmonary damage
- Promoting recovery of the lungs, when possible
- Treating the associated underlying condition(s)

Blood Oxygenation. The most immediate, life-threatening problem in ARDS is inadequate tissue oxygen delivery. This is treated first with mechanical ventilatory support and supplemental oxygen. The equipment and methods required include a cuffed endotracheal tube or tracheostomy; a volume-cycled ventilator; precise control of inspired oxygen concentration; and the application of positive end-expiratory pressure (PEEP).

Initially, high concentrations of *oxygen* (F_{IO_2}) in the range of 0.5–1.0 (50–100%) may be needed. These levels are toxic to the lungs when administered for prolonged periods of time; hence, they should be reduced as soon as possible, compatible with maintenance of adequate tissue oxygenation. The use of PEEP allows a reduction of F_{IO_2}. In combination with PEEP, choose the lowest F_{IO_2} necessary to maintain adequate tissue oxygenation. This is achieved when the hemoglobin saturation (Sa_{O_2}) is 90%, which usually occurs when the Pa_{O_2} is about 60 mm Hg. Achieving a Pa_{O_2} above 60 mm Hg adds little to the oxygen content of the blood or to tissue oxygenation and unnecessarily increases the risk of oxygen toxicity. Using an F_{IO_2} above 0.50 for prolonged periods of time should be avoided. Hyperbaric oxygen is not useful in the treatment of ARDS.

The management of *assisted mechanical ventilation* is reviewed in detail in Chapter 16. For ARDS, an initial tidal volume of 10–12 ml/kg of ideal body weight is preferred. However, this must be adjusted according to lung compliance measurements in order to reduce the risk of barotrauma. The assist–control mode of ventilation should be used. A patient-initiated respiratory rate is preferable, but proper ventilation may require totally controlled mechanical ventilation when the patient is struggling or when hyperventilation with respiratory alkalosis is a problem. Sedation of the patient and paralysis with pancuronium bromide (pavulon) may need to be used to achieve total control. Pancuronium does not affect consciousness; hence, it is essential to use a concomitant sedative in the awake patient. Intermittent mandatory ventilation may be deleterious in the management of acute ARDS (by increasing oxygen demand) and it should be avoided.

PEEP generally improves gas exchange across the lung and is almost always needed to treat ARDS. Since PEEP has serious dose-related side effects, including reduced cardiac output and tissue oxygen delivery, it is best to use levels no higher than 5–15 cm H_2O and to monitor cardiac output and $S\bar{v}_{O_2}$ as well as ABG. Choose the lowest level that allows reduction of the $F_{I_{O_2}}$ to less than 0.6 while still providing adequate tissue oxygenation ($S\bar{v}_{O_2} > 70\%$).

Perfusion and Tissue Oxygenation. The measurement and optimization of tissue oxygen uptake requires Swan–Ganz catheterization for measurement of cardiac output ($\dot{Q}$), pulmonary capillary wedge pressure (Ppcw), and mixed venous oxygen saturation ($S\bar{v}_{O_2}$). It also requires arterial catheterization for monitoring ABGs and mean arterial pressure (MAP). Determination of the arteriovenous oxygen content difference is a valuable indicator of tissue oxygen delivery. A fall in mixed venous oxygen saturation ($S\bar{v}_{O_2}$) and a rise in arterial–venous oxygen difference usually indicates inadequate oxygen delivery, which may be due to low hemoglobin, low Sa_{O_2}, or low cardiac output ($\dot{Q}$). It may mean that PEEP must be reduced and $F_{I_{O_2}}$ increased to maintain Sa_{O_2} and improve $\dot{Q}$. (Unfortunately, the converse is not necessarily true; normal or improving values for these parameters do not guarantee that there is adequate oxygen delivery to tissues or adequate tissue utilization of the oxygen delivered.)

Careful *fluid management* is critical to the proper management of ARDS (Table 7). Fluid administration should be adjusted to maintain adequate circulation and perfusion (as reflected in adequate MAP, CO, and $S\bar{v}_{O_2}$) while at the same time avoiding overload (reflected in rising Ppcw), which would lead to increased fluid sequestration in the lung. In general, Ppcw should be reduced as low as is compatible with maintenance of adequate cardiac output and tissue perfusion. At times, reducing the Ppcw may require the use of diuretics (furosemide), vasodilators (sodium nitroprusside), and/or restriction of fluids.

When low cardiac output is associated with ARDS, inotropic agents (digitalis, dopamine) may be needed; a combination of inotropic agents and peripheral vasodilators (nitroprusside) for unloading may improve tissue perfusion and oxygen delivery in some circumstances.

Crystalloid solutions are preferred for fluid volume replacement in ARDS, when needed. If anemia is present, red cells should be transfused to optimize the blood's oxygen content.

In general, optimum therapy from the point of view of tissue perfusion and oxygenation involves achievement of the lowest possible levels of PEEP, $F_{I_{O_2}}$, and Ppcw sufficient to maintain adequate circulation ($\dot{Q}$ and

TABLE 7. Management of ARDS in the Intensive Care Unit[a]

Recommended monitoring
  Hemodynamics (Swan–Ganz catheter and arterial line)—Ppa, Ppcw, $\dot{Q}$, $S\bar{v}_{O_2}$, MAP, EKG, Hb, Ca-$\bar{v}_{O_2}$
  Respiratory parameters (mechanical ventilator, arterial line)—C, T.V., R.R., P_{aw}, V_D/V_T, ABG
Mechanical ventilation
  Endotracheal intubation
  Volume-cycled ventilator (10–12 cc/kg tidal volume initially)
  Assist–control mode (avoid IMV in acute phase)
  PEEP 5–15 cm H_2O (sufficient for Pa_{O_2} 60 with $F_{I_{O_2}}$ < 0.6)
Oxygen therapy
  50–100% (0.5–1.0 $F_{I_{O_2}}$) initially
  <50% as early as possible
  Goal is Pa_{O_2} 60
Fluid management
  Crystalloid intravenous fluids
  Goal is Ppcw < 12 mm Hg with MAP > 70 mm Hg and $S\bar{v}_{O_2}$ > 70%
  Diuretics for Ppcw > 12 mm Hg if $\dot{Q}$ and MAP adequate
  Inotropic agents for low cardiac output (first rule out PEEP effect)
Other measures
  Corticosteroids
  Antacids or cimetidine
  Prophylactic heparin (if no bleeding contraindication)
  Nutritional support
  Aseptic technique
  Prophylaxis for pressure necrosis

---

[a] Ppa = pulmonary artery pressure; Ppcw = pulmonary capillary wedge pressure; $\dot{Q}$ = cardiac output; $S\bar{v}_{O_2}$ = mixed venous oxygen saturation; Hb = hemoglobin; Ca-$\bar{v}_{O_2}$ = arteriovenous oxygen content difference; MAP = mean arterial pressure; EKG = electrocardiogram; C = lung compliance; T.V. = tidal volume; R.R. = respiratory rate; Paw = airway pressure; V_D/V_T = fraction of dead space volume in tidal volume; ABG = arterial blood gas; PEEP = positive end-expiratory pressure; $F_{I_{O_2}}$ = fraction of inspired oxygen.

MAP) and tissue oxygenation ($S\bar{v}_{O_2}$), using mechanical ventilation, supplemental oxygen, fluids, blood, diuresis, inotropic agents, and vasodilators.

Promoting Lung Recovery. Additional measures that may promote lung recovery include the following:

- Corticosteroids: Although still controversial, methylprednisolone (or equivalent) may be given intravenously, 30 mg/kg at 4–8-hr intervals for up to 48 hr. Treat associated glucose intolerance with insulin if necessary.
- Nutritional support: Early parenteral hyperalimentation is frequently needed.
- Antibiotics: Use only for definite or probable infection. Prophylactic use is not warranted.
- Treat the underlying disease process.

Other Measures. Additional general measures that will prevent complications include the following:

- Antacid or cimetidine therapy to prevent stress ulcers
- Low-dose subcutaneous heparin to prevent venous thrombosis and possible pulmonary emboli
- Meticulous attention to aseptic technique (hand washing, equipment sterilization, intravenous lines, urinary catheter care, airway care) to reduce infection
- Special attention to prevention of pressure necrosis, e.g., using sheepskin or air mattress, taping and padding endotracheal and nasogastric tubes

BIBLIOGRAPHY

1. Albert RL: Pulmonary edema, in Sahn SA (ed): *Pulmonary Emergencies.* New York, Churchill, Livingstone, 1982, p. 149.
2. Braunwald E: Heart failure, in Petersdorf R, et al (eds): *Harrison's Principles of Internal Medicine,* ed 10. New York, McGraw-Hill, 1983, p 1353.
3. Brigham KL: Mechanisms of lung injury. *Clin Chest Med* 3:9, 1982.
4. Deneke SM, Fanburg BL: Normobaric oxygen toxicity of the lung. *N Engl J Med* 303:76, 1980.
5. Fein AM, Goldberg SK, Walkenstein MD: Is pulmonary artery catheterization necessary for the diagnosis of pulmonary edema? *Am Rev Respir Dis* 129:1006, 1984.
6. Fisher HK, Clements JA, Wright RK: Enhancement of oxygen toxicity by the herbicide paraquat, *Am Rev Respir Dis* 107:246, 1973.
7. Fowler AA, Hammon RF, Good JT: Risk of the adult respiratory distress syndrome following common predispositions. *Ann Intern Med* 98:553, 1983.
8. Gong H: Positive pressure ventilation in the adult respiratory distress syndrome. *Clin Chest Med* 3:69, 1982.
9. Hudson LD: Ventilatory management of patients with adult respiratory distress syndrome. *Semin Respir Med* 2:128, 1981.
10. Jardin F, Farciet JC, Boisante L: Influence of positive end-expiratory pressure on left ventricular performance. *N Engl J Med* 304:387, 1981.
11. Pierson DJ, Hudson LD: Monitoring hemodynamics in the critically ill. *Med Clin North Am* 67:1343, 1983.
12. Sahn AN, Forrester JS, Waters DD: Hospital treatment of congestive heart failure. *Am J Med* 65:173, 1978.
13. Tate RM, Petty TL: Primary pulmonary edema. *Adv Intern Med* 29:471, 1984.
14. Wood LH, Pruitt RM: Cardiovascular management in acute hypoxemic respiratory failure. *Am J Cardiol* 47:963, 1981.

CHAPTER 7

Near-Drowning

Kenneth Dickie

Drowning is the flooding of the living, intact airway with a liquid. It commonly occurs in healthy persons by accidental aspiration of fresh, brackish, or seawater, during recreational activities. If the process results in death, the person is said to be "drowned," or if interrupted prior to death, "near-drowned," hence the term "near-drowning."

Drowning consists of a series of events: panic, maximal exertion with hyperventilation, exhaustion, submersion with immediate breath holding, swallowing of large quantities of water, vomiting, involuntary gasping, flooding of the lungs, and death. Death is also reported to occur with prolonged submersion of the airway without flooding. Most drownings occur within 10 yards of the shore in large bodies of water, or in swimming pools. About two-thirds are in fresh water and at least a third have alcohol intoxication as a factor. A sizable proportion have associated problems such as prior seizure activity; traumatic injury due to swimming pool, boating, or auto accidents; body and airway burns, with smoke inhalation; and sometimes, decompression sickness, air embolism, and/or hypothermia. Often, medical care is not sought because the drowning is interrupted prior to impairing the airways, or the effects are minor and completely reversible without assistance. Unfortunately, the other extreme is also common, the process proceeds too far and the victim dies before assistance is possible. This discussion concerns the patient between these extremes.

By definition, the history will contain evidence that airway submersion may have occurred. The history is the primary component in problem recognition, but it may not be sufficient. The involuntary submersion and aspiration may not have been observed, and particularly in alcohol-related accidents, the patient may not remember the event clearly.

Kenneth Dickie • Division of Pulmonary Diseases and Allergy, George Washington University School of Medicine and Health Sciences, Washington, D.C. 20037; Veterans Administration Medical Center, Washington, D.C. 20422.

The following information will assist in assessing the problem:

- Extent of the drowning
- Resuscitation methods used or attempted
- Medications given since the accident
- Response of the patient since the accident
- Cardiac or respiratory support given during resuscitation
- Associated trauma, smoke inhalation, or airway burn
- Prior medication including nonprescribed alcohol and drugs
- Prior medical status, including seizure history

DIFFERENTIAL DIAGNOSIS

Drowning is primarily established by history. In the absence of a history, the nonspecific findings of cough, dyspnea, rales, and wheezes, a "whitening" of the lung fields on chest x ray, and hypoxia, could be confused for any of the causes of acute respiratory distress syndrome (see Chapter 6). The circumstances in which drowning occurs almost always raise the possibility of drowning, but it may be difficult to determine that drowning actually occurred. The primary problem may be inebriation and exhaustion, which does not require treatment for drowning. Alternately, the objective signs of drowning, such as the chest x ray and arterial blood gas abnormalities, may be delayed, and the diagnosis may be missed, or underestimated in severity, unless the patient is observed for a period of time.

The history of near-drowning may lead to a considerable overestimate of the brain damage and the bleakness of the prognosis. There are reports of patient survival, without brain damage, after 30 min of submersion. This long survival has several possible explanations. The more common, heart-initiated, cardiopulmonary arrest results in an instant, complete cessation of delivery of nutrients to the brain, which results in brain death in a few minutes. Drowning usually occurs in water that is below body temperature, thereby reducing the metabolic needs of the body, while the cardiovascular system continues to provide nutrients to the brain after respiration has ceased; this may account for the prolonged brain viability. Other explanations for prolonged survival include the protection given by the diving reflex, the physiologic response to hypothermia, or simply that during the excitement of the drowning the time is inaccurately estimated.

A near-drowned patient with altered mental status, decreased alertness, agitation, combativeness, or coma may have permanent neurologic damage. Neurologic deficits that persist, or increase, may indicate other head injury, such as subdural hematoma, which may require different treatment, and should be investigated. Recent reports of pediatric intensive neurologic care shows that survival from brain damage due to drowning is possible, with little or no permanent neurologic defect.

PROBLEM ASSESSMENT

Initial History

Determine that water was or may have been aspirated, and whether or not there is a need for emergency therapy. Severe respiratory distress requires immediate physical and laboratory assessment and emergency therapy. Once the necessary emergency measures have been started, the following data should be obtained:

Activities that preceded the drowning
- Diving to depth
- Alcohol intake
- Previous history of seizures
- Prior illness or disease, particularly of the lung

The submersion that occurred
- Type of water (fresh treated or natural, sea, brackish)
- Length of time of submersion
- Likelihood of water aspiration

Complications during the drowning
- Trauma—particularly to neck
- Burns or smoke inhalation
- Aspiration of water contaminants

Resuscitation that was necessary and/or attempted
- Type and extent of resuscitation
- Immediate response
- Course of response
- Vomiting—possible aspiration of gastric contents
- Seizure activity during resuscitation

Initial Physical Examination and Laboratory Tests

The clinical examination should be adjusted to the condition of the patient and to the available facilities. This tasking outline must be modified as experience and circumstances require.

If the patient is awake and alert without symptoms

1. Measure respiratory rate, pulse, blood pressure, and temperature.
2. Examine the chest, including the heart.
3. Measure arterial blood gases and pH.

If the patient has respiratory, cardiovascular, or neurologic symptoms

1. Give oxygen by mask.
2. Measure arterial oxygen, carbon dioxide, and pH.
3. Measure respiratory rate, pulse, blood pressure, and temperature.
4. Measure serum sodium, chloride, potassium, and carbon dioxide.
5. Measure serum magnesium (if available, for sea- or brackish water).
6. Measure white blood count, hemoglobin, hematocrit.
7. Obtain and immediately read a chest x ray.
8. Obtain and immediately read an electrocardiogram.
9. Send a specimen for urinalysis.
10. Complete a neurologic examination including
    a. Ocular reflexes,
    b. State of consciousness,
    c. Motor response to stimuli
    d. Verbal command response.

PARAMETERS TO BE FOLLOWED

Table 1 summarizes the clinical and laboratory expectations in near-drowning. The presenting clinical findings vary from the mild complex of cough, tachypnea, and perhaps shortness of breath, to severe distress with fulminant pulmonary edema requiring respiratory assistance. One-third of patients may require intubation and mechanical ventilatory assistance, with gradual recovery expected over 48–72 hr. Longer periods of persistent respiratory distress, failure, and decreased lung compliance may indicate complications. Severe cardiopulmonary symptoms may occur after several hours have lapsed, so all patients with submersion should be observed for several hours.

THERAPEUTIC MANAGEMENT

The therapy for patients with drowning is summarized in Fig. 1. It can be divided into three categories.

TABLE 1. Clinical Findings and Expectations in Near-Drowning

Examination	Finding	Significance
Temperature	38°C < 24 hr	Expected
	38°C > 24 hr	Look for infection
	<33°C	Monitor closely
	<28°C	Risk of ventricular fibrillation
	<25°C	Risk of shock
Upper airways	Foreign material	Remove
Lungs	Normal	Expected
	Few rales	May be pulmonary edema
	Fulminant lung edema	ARDS
Neurologic	Normal	Expected
	Abnormal	Severe problem Intensive care required
	Decreased alertness, agitation, combativeness, or coma	Trauma, alcohol, or drug— may be hypoxic cortical necrosis with reduced prognosis
Chest x ray	Normal	Expected 1 in 4
	Infiltrates	Clear in 24–48 hr
	Generalized dense edema	Clear in 72–96 hr
	Persistent infiltrates	Chemical pneumonitis, infection, atelectasis
EKG	Normal	Expected
	Supraventricular arrhythmias	Common—transient
P_{O_2}	Normal	Expected
	Reduced	Increase $F_{I_{O_2}}$ Look for metabolic or respiratory acidosis
P_{CO_2}	Elevated	Usually transient
	Low	Hyperventilating Look for hypoxia
	Increasing	May be normalizing or developing respiratory failure
pH	Normal	Expected
	Decreased	Metabolic acidosis Respiratory component
Blood alcohol	May be elevated	Prior consumption
Electrolytes	Sodium and chloride elevated	Expected for 1 hr
	Magnesium elevated	Seawater aspiration
Blood volume		
Fresh water	Hypervolemia	Initial
	Hypovolemia	Within 1 hr
Salt water	Hypovolemia	Initial
	Normal	About 1–2 hr
White blood count	Up to 40,000	24–48 hr
Hemoglobin	Predrowning value	Usual
Hematocrit	Reduced	Occasional
Urinalysis	Normal	Expected
	Hemoglobin	Occasional for hours

- Observation only
- Temporary assistance while problems resolve
- Major support

Category I: Observation Only

These patients are asymptomatic after an accidental episode of sub-mersion, but have probable or certain aspiration without subjective or objective pathologic findings. The vital signs, chest auscultation, arterial blood gases, and chest x ray are normal.

Actions. Repeat vital signs and chest auscultation in 30 min and then hourly, from 4 to 8 hr. (Acute symptoms may begin 8 hr after submersion.) If the examinations continue to be normal, release the patient from observation.

If clinical abnormalities develop, handle the patient as in category II.

Cateogry II: Abnormalities Are Present, but Not Severe

Give oxygen and re-examine the patient in 15 min and then every 30 min for 4 hr. If the examinations are negative after 4 hr, decrease the frequency of the observations, but continue to observe the patient for 24 hr. Measure arterial blood gases and pH if symptoms or examination findings change and modify therapy appropriately (see oxygen therapy below). If abnormality increases, follow category III.

Category III: Major Support Is, or May Be, Required

These patients present with symptoms and/or other clinical abnormalities:

Hypoxia. An arterial blood oxygen measurement that is less than normal indicates the need for supplemental airway oxygen. The level of oxygen in the blood is related to airway concentration of oxygen but is also affected by the ventilation–perfusion relationships, cardiac output, and peripheral extraction. These will change during therapy and are only partially subject to therapeutic control. Therefore, it is necessary to mea-sure arterial blood gases each time the clinical status of the patient changes. Arterial blood should be maintained 90% saturated with oxygen, while using the least possible fractional airway oxygen. Balancing the need to maintain high oxygen saturation while keeping the possibility of

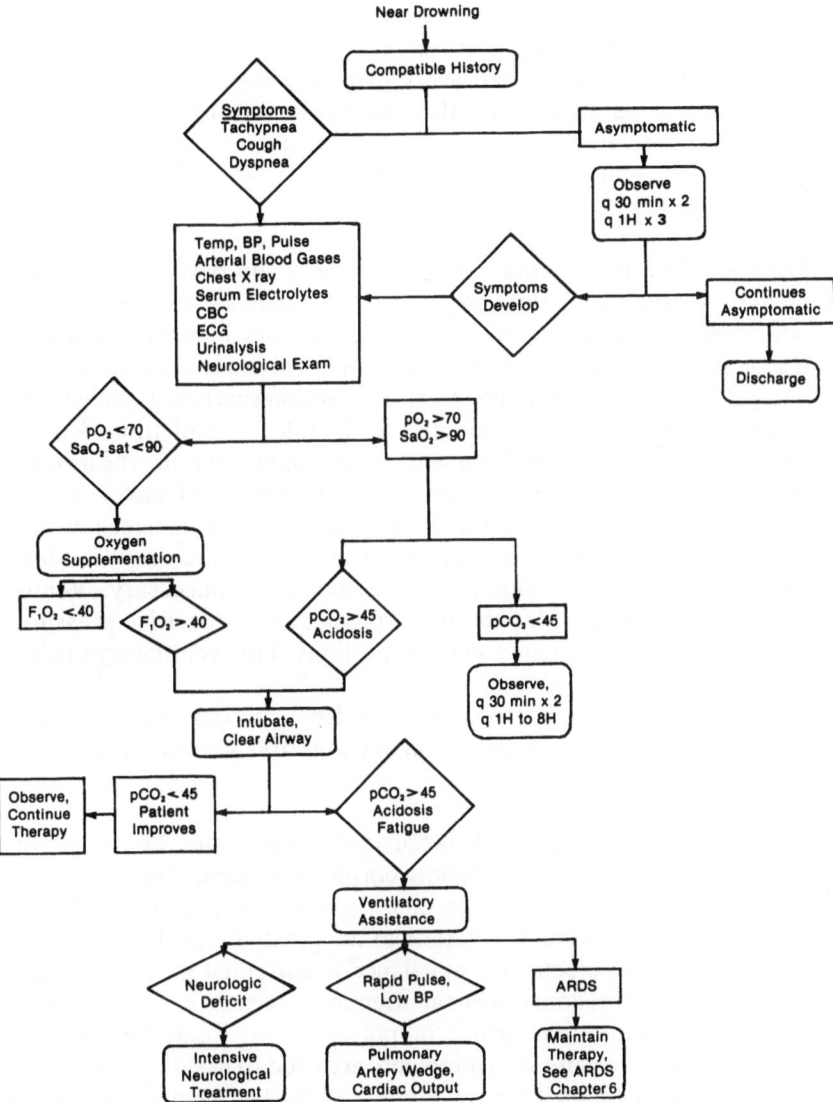

FIGURE 1. Algorithm for evaluation and management of near-drowning.

toxicity low is frequently difficult. Acute short-term therapy, maintaining the blood oxygen at 100 Torr, will assist in reversing the hypoxia in the tissues. After 24 hr, if not sooner, a lower level, 70 Torr, should be maintained to prevent acidosis while reducing the risk of oxygen toxicity.

An endotracheal tube may be necessary to supply a high concentration of oxygen, to provide a route for suctioning the patient's airway, or to mechanically support ventilation.

Assisted ventilation, using large tidal volumes or maintaining a positive end-expired pressure, will increase the alveolar participation in ventilation and may decrease the necessary fractional inspired oxygen. Oxygenation will also be affected by the changes in the fluid balance that occur in these patients. Central venous, pulmonary artery, pulmonary capillary wedge pressures, and cardiac outputs may be needed to evaluate the status of these patients.

Hypoventilation. Arterial carbon dioxide is the best clinical measurement of ventilation. Below-normal readings indicate excess, normal indicates adequate, and a high carbon dioxide level indicates deficient ventilation (assuming no significant metabolic acid–base abnormality).

For patients in respiratory distress, an increasing carbon dioxide level rising above normal indicates the need for increased ventilation. Ventilation may improve by reducing the work of breathing; clearing the airway of obstruction using bronchodilators; removing aspirated material and secretions; reducing the compliance of the lung by fluid management or by supplementing the airway oxygen. If these methods are unsuccessful, intubation and mechanical ventilatory assistance are necessary. Ventilatory assistance can provide rate, tidal volume, and/or positive pressure control of the airway throughout selected portions of the ventilatory cycle.

Vomiting. If vomiting is occurring, or has occurred, and the respiratory system appears endangered, insert a gastric suction catheter to empty the stomach.

Fluids. The electrolyte imbalance initiated by salt-, brackish-, or fresh-water drowning is usually rapidly corrected without therapy. In experimental animals, blood volume expansion occurs within 3 min of fresh-water aspirations and is back to less than the prestudy level within 1 hr. In most patients, the electrolyte imbalance is corrected by the time the patient receives professional medical attention. Occasionally, abnormalities of blood volume and cardiac output are seen. Central venous or pulmonary wedge pressure measurements are used to assess the need for fluid control to maintain cardiac output. Persistent electrolyte abnormalities suggest that another disorder is present.

Hypothermia. Intragastric balloons, colonic irrigations, peritoneal dialysis, and hemodialysis are used for rewarming. Medications given to the patient while hypothermic may accumulate at the low temperatures and become active as temperature is raised. Complications of overdosage may then become apparent.

Neurologic. Intensive neurologic therapy may prevent some of the neurologic complications of drowning and will reduce the residual neurologic disorder in other patients. An outline of therapy for children in deep coma is given here, but the original references should be consulted for details (see Pfenninger and Sutter in Bibliography). The principles of therapy are hyperventilation, fluid restriction, and diuretics, corticosteroids, and barbiturates.

Hyperventilation. Use nasotracheal intubation with muscle relaxation and artificial ventilation to maintain Pa_{O_2} at 100–150 mm Hg and Pa_{CO_2} at 25–30 mm Hg. If intracranial pressure is persistently elevated, maintain Pa_{CO_2} at 15–20 mm Hg.

Body Temperature. Maintain temperature at 35.5°–36.5°C rectal using cooling, chlorpromazine, and muscle relaxants. If the intracranial pressure is significantly increased, lower body temperature to 30°C.

Fluids. Keep the patient in a slightly negative fluid balance (Ppcw < 8, output + insensible loss > intake) using furosemide, 0.5–1 mg/kg body weight, and mannitol, 0.3–5 g/kg body weight.

Dexamethasone. Give 1–1.5 mg/kg per day intravenously in six to eight divided doses (initial dose of 1–1.5 mg/kg).

Mean Arterial Pressure. Maintain in normal–low normal range by intravenous dopamine or intravascular volume contraction as necessary.

Barbiturates. A recent randomized clinical study of comatose survivors of cardiac arrest, who may have had similar cerebral damage as drowning victims but differ in age and initiating cause of the cerebral insult, did not find any advantage to using thiopental loading. This indicates that barbiturate loading is not a significant factor in preventing long term neurologic damage.

OTHER INJURIES OR MEDICAL COMPLICATIONS ASSOCIATED WITH DROWNING

- Acute renal failure, reported in rare instances, appears to be prevented by maintaining adequate fluid volume
- Increased permeability pulmonary edema, pneumonia, lung abscess, and empyema.
- Injuries during resuscitation such as pneumothorax and pneumomediastinum
- Seizures, especially during resuscitation
- Cerebral edema
- Severe hemorrhagic disorder
- Air embolism and decompression sickness associated with scuba diving

BIBLIOGRAPHY

1. Harries MG: Drowning in man. *Crit Care Med* 9:407–408, 1981.
2. Modell JH: *Pathophysiology and Treatment of Drowning and Near-Drowning.* Springfield, IL, Charles C Thomas, 1971.
3. Pfenninger J, Sutter M: Intensive care after fresh water immersion accidents in children. *Anaesthesia* 37:1157–1162, 1982.
4. Redding JS: Drowning and near-drowning. Can the victim be saved? *Postgrad Med* 74:85–97, 1983.
5. Tabeling BB, Modell JH: Fluid administration increases oxygen delivery during continuous positive pressure ventilation after fresh water near-drowning. *Crit Care Med* 11:693–696, 1983.
6. Brain Resusitation Clinical Trial I Study Group: Randomized clinical study of thiopental loading in comatose survivers of cardiac arrest. *N Engl J Med* 314:397–402, 1986.

CHAPTER 8

Chest Trauma

Truvor Kuzmowych

A physician is much more likely to see patients with blunt (or closed) chest trauma than with penetrating chest injuries, unless he works in a trauma center or in the emergency room of a major metropolitan hospital. Patients with chest injuries are frequently in critical condition and require rapid diagnosis with institution of prompt therapy. Emergency thoracotomy, however, is needed in approximately 10% of patients with major chest trauma.

The most common cause of *blunt* chest trauma is injury sustained in automobile accidents. Other important causes include falls from great heights, blast or crush injuries, airplane crashes, cave ins, and contact sport accidents. Thoracic injuries resulting from blunt chest trauma are listed in Table 1. The discussion of blunt chest trauma in this chapter is limited primarily to chest wall injuries, injury to the pulmonary parenchyma, disruption of the mediastinum, and diaphragmatic injuries. Traumatic disruption of the pleural space is discussed in Chapter 15.

Cardiovascular injuries resulting from blunt chest trauma are extremely serious and quite common occurrences. However, they will not be discussed in this chapter.

EMERGENCY EVALUATION AND GENERAL GUIDELINES

In the initial evaluation of any patient with trauma, the "ABC's" must be observed: A—airway, B—breathing, C—circulatory system.

Truvor Kuzmowych • Division of Pulmonary Diseases and Allergy, George Washington University School of Medicine and Health Sciences, Washington, D.C. 20037; Pulmonary Clinic, Veterans Administration Medical Center, Washington, D.C. 20422.

TABLE 1. Thoracic Injuries Resulting from Blunt
Chest Trauma

1. Chest wall injuries
    a. Chest wall contusions
    b. Clavicular fractures
    c. Rib fractures
    d. Flail chest
    e. Sternal fractures
2. Disruption of the pleural space
    a. Pneumothorax
    b. Hemothorax
    c. Chylothorax
3. Injuries of the pulmonary parenchyma
    a. Pulmonary contusion
    b. Hematoma of the lung
    c. Pulmonary laceration
    d. Tracheobronchial injuries
4. Disruption of the mediastinum
    a. Pneumomediastinum
    b. Rupture of the esophagus
5. Cardiovascular injuries
    a. Injuries of the heart and pericardium
    b. Rupture of the aorta
    c. Injury of the innominate and/or subclavian arteries
6. Diaphragmatic rupture

A. The airway must be kept patent. When a cervical fracture is suspected, the neck should be stabilized. The oropharynx must be examined to remove foreign bodies and/or dentures. When suspected, mandibular fractures or laryngeal trauma should be ruled out.

B. Once the airway is clear, it is important to determine whether the patient is breathing properly. This is done by examining the trachea to see if it is in the midline, determining whether the chest wall is moving symmetrically with respiration, and noting whether parts of the chest wall are out of synchrony with respiration. Determine, by percussion, whether hyperresonance or dullness is present over the chest area. Determine, by auscultation, whether air is entering both lungs. Observe for wounds or discoloration on the chest wall.

C. Once it is clearly established that the patient is ventilating properly, immediate assessment of the circulatory system should be undertaken. The heart rate, blood pressure, as well as the quality of the heart sounds, and pattern of pulse should be noted. The presence of pulses in each extremity and the appearance of the neck veins should be observed. The texture, color, and warmth of the patient's skin should also be noted.

After establishing the initial baseline information, and barring the need for immediate cardiopulmonary resuscitation, proceed quickly to obtain a history and perform a thorough physical examination. Then, after initiating any immediate resuscitative measures (establishing a large-bore i.v. route and/or supplemental oxygen), diagnostic tests should be obtained. Choose tests that will most effectively provide a definitive diagnosis and expose the patient to the least amount of risk. Obtain consultations from the cardiothoracic and/or trauma surgeons early.

CHEST WALL CONTUSIONS

Chest wall contusions present clinically as areas of tenderness and/or ecchymosis over the chest wall. A mild degree of swelling and/or induration may also be present. Chest wall contusion alone is usually not a serious injury. It can be managed with mild, nonnarcotic analgesics. However, if the force causing the contusion is severe, complications can arise from associated intrathoracic injuries despite the absence of rib fractures. This is especially common in children and young athletes with flexible rib cages and in people exposed to underwater blast injuries. A careful history and physical examination, including a chest x ray, must be done to identify such complications.

CLAVICULAR FRACTURES

Clavicular fractures can result from an indirect force applied to the clavicle, such as a blow to the shoulder or a fall on an outstretched arm. More commonly, in blunt chest trauma, the clavicle is fractured by a direct force; for example, collision with a steering wheel or the dashboard of an automobile. The clinical signs of clavicular fractures vary from tenderness over the clavicle to an open wound with bone fragments protruding. When bone fragments are displaced, there may be shortening of the distance between the base of the neck and the tip of the shoulder joint on the involved side. Diagnosis of clavicular fracture depends on a careful examination of the upper anterior chest. It is confirmed by a posteroanterior (PA) and cross-table lateral x ray centered on the clavicle. A nondisplaced clavicular fracture, occurring lateral to the coracoclavicular ligament, may be treated symptomatically with a sling. Fractures medial to the coracoclavicular ligament are treated with a well-applied clavicular strap. If the fracture is linear and without displacement, a figure-of-eight splint may be used. For more serious and complicated fractures, surgical fixation may be required. Acute complications of clavicular fractures include pneumothorax and/or fractures of the ipsilateral first two ribs. Excess callus formation may result in brachial plexus symptoms or thoracic-outlet syndrome.

RIB FRACTURES

Rib fractures are the most common injury resulting from chest trauma. The ribs lose their resiliency with age and become more brittle. In elderly people "minor" bumps may produce rib fractures. The fifth to ninth ribs are most frequently fractured. Much less common are fractures of the first four ribs. Fractures of these ribs are usually caused by an extremely violent force and are, therefore, frequently associated with concomitant injury to the thoracic aorta and major bronchi or disruption of the neurovascular structures in the upper extremity. The point of fracture of a rib depends on the amount, direction, and distribution of the force applied to the chest. A well-concentrated blow to the chest results in a rib fracture at the point of contact. An intense force applied over a large area of the chest results in multiple rib fractures and may also fracture ribs in the area of the chest wall opposite to the area of impact.

Symptoms and Signs

The patient usually complains of point tenderness on the chest wall made worse by deep breathing. Skin discoloration is usually absent. If the fracture fragments are displaced, bone crepitation may be felt by the examiner.

Although there may be no underlying damage to the lung tissue, rib fractures frequently diminish ventilation because of pain. Breathing is shallow, and atelectasis often develops. This may lead to impaired gas exchange and/or pneumonia, especially in the elderly and in individuals with reduced lung function.

X rays of the ribs with PA and right and left oblique views of the chest usually confirm the diagnosis. Chest x rays should be taken in both inspiration and exhalation to detect any associated pneumothorax.

Management

As a general rule, it is advisable to hospitalize patients with two or more rib fractures for a period of 24–48 hr of observation. This is especially important if the ninth, tenth, or eleventh ribs are involved. In such lower-rib-cage fractures, the possibility of associated hepatic and/or splenic injury is increased. These injuries may not be evident until several hours following the injury. When seven or more rib fractures are present, there is a 60–70% incidence of associated internal thoracic injury, as well as a 20% incidence of intra-abdominal associated injury. For this reason, should a patient with rib fractures develop sudden hypotension without evidence of a pneumothorax or hemothorax, intra-abdominal bleeding must be immediately suspected and investigated.

External Support. Strapping rib fractures with adhesive tape is usually of little value and may be harmful by further limiting respiration and inducing atelectasis. When external support is used, a rib belt permits easier management and less skin trauma.

Analgesia. Chest wall pain from rib fractures is best managed with the judicious use of mild narcotics, such as codeine, 30–60 mg every 3–4 hr. This dose does not usually oversuppress the patient's cough reflex; however, the patient should be instructed to take frequent (every hour) deep breaths.

Intercostal Block. For severe pain, or for multiple rib fractures, intercostal nerve block with 1–5 ml of 2% lidocaine (or a longer-acting local anesthetic) can be used. The total dose of lidocaine should not exceed 7–10 mg/kg of body weight. Intercostal nerve block provides relief of pain and is effective for 4–6 hr, at which time it may be repeated. A chest x ray should be obtained following intercostal nerve block to evaluate the possibility of an iatrogenic pneumothorax.

FLAIL CHEST

Segmental rib fractures (fractures in two or more locations on the same rib) of three or more ribs result in instability of the chest wall. This instability, or flail, is characterized by paradoxic inward movement of a segment of the chest wall during inspiration. Instability may be present in the anterior, posterior, or lateral chest wall. The most common location is the lateral flail chest.

The anterior flail chest is frequently associated with a costochondral separation and/or transverse sternal fracture. The breathing pattern in an anterior flail is like a seesaw; i.e., the chest wall sinks in as the abdominal wall goes out on inspiration.

The posterior flail chest is the most difficult to recognize because the sacrospinalis muscles and scapula splint the chest wall, reducing the paradox of the unstable segment. Also, on inspiration, the posterior excursion of the chest wall is less than the anterior portion, making the flail more subtle.

Loss of stability of the chest wall results in loss of the ability to generate sufficient negative intrapleural pressure to fully expand the lungs on inspiration. This loss of efficiency of the bellows action of the chest wall, combined with the associated damage to the underlying lung, and hypoventilation secondary to splinting as a result of chest pain are the three main causes for the development of respiratory failure in patients with flail chest. The diagnosis of flail chest may be initially overlooked, especially if the unstable segment is small, posterior in location, and accompanied by muscle splinting and/or tissue swelling. Frequently, only when breathing becomes more difficult for the patient does the flail become more obvious.

Treatment

Although many techniques have been devised in the past to stabilize the thorax in flail chest, current therapy consists of one of the following:

- Splinting the chest wall externally by use of sandbags
- Internal splinting of the chest wall by means of endotracheal intubation and mechanical ventilation
- Open reduction and internal fixation of the ribs with Kirschner wires

Placing a sandbag over the flail segment is an effective temporary measure to stabilize the chest wall and improve ventilation, as is turning the patient over with the injured side down, or just pressing firmly with the hand against the paradoxic portion of the chest wall. However, a flail chest is rarely an isolated injury to the chest wall. The most commonly associated injury, and one that is frequently overlooked, is pulmonary contusion (see below). In addition, flail chest in the presence of seven or more rib fractures, shock, head trauma, intra-abdominal injuries, skeletal fractures, myocardial contusion, or age over 60, has a significantly increased mortality. Early intubation and mechanical ventilation may be beneficial in the prevention of fulminant respiratory failure in flail chest with any of the above associated injuries, and thus improve survival.

Open reduction and internal fixation of rib fractures with Kirschner wires is effective but requires general anesthesia and should be reserved for those patients who require a thoracotomy for exploration and repair of underlying lung damage.

STERNAL FRACTURES

Sternal fracture is a serious injury produced by severe trauma. Table 2 lists other commonly associated injuries. The majority of the fractures occur in the body of the sternum near its junction with the manubrium.

TABLE 2. Injuries Commonly associated with Sternal
Fractures

Flail chest	Cardiac injuries
Pulmonary contusion	Ruptured thoracic aorta
Tracheobronchial rupture	Abdominal visceral injuries
Hemo- and/or pneumothorax	Spinal injuries
Pericardial injuries	

Sternal fractures produce pain over the sternum that is aggravated by coughing or deep breathing. There may be skin discoloration over the fracture site, overriding of the fracture fragments, swelling, crepitation, and tenderness to palpation over the sternum. Occasionally an undisplaced sternal fracture is asymptomatic. Diagnosis is confirmed on lateral or oblique chest x rays. Conservative symptomatic therapy for pain is usually all that is required for a simple sternal fracture. Surgical fixation or reconstructive surgery may be needed for severely displaced or open fractures.

PULMONARY CONTUSION

Pulmonary contusion is defined as traumatic lung parenchymal injury with edema and hemorrhage occurring in the absence of laceration of lung tissue. Lung contusion is commonly associated with blunt chest trauma and has a reported mortality of up to 40%.

The basic phenomenon involved in the etiology of pulmonary contusion is a combination of the spalling effect, the implosion effect, and the inertial effect. The spalling effect is the destructive phenomenon seen when a shock wave moving in a liquid encounters a gas–liquid interface. As the shock wave is partially transmitted into the gas, energy is released and the interface (the alveolar–capillary membrane) is disrupted. The implosion effect is the rebound, or overexpansion, occurring in bubbles after a positive pressure (overpressure) wave passes. Such an effect can diffusely rip pulmonary paraenchyma by stretching it too far or too quickly. The inertial effect occurs as low-density aleveolar tissue is stripped from the hilar structures when they are accelerated at varying rates by a shock wave. It is important to note that lethal shock waves can be effectively generated in the lung without having to perforate, or even seriously damage, the chest wall.

The pathologic changes found in lung contusion include alveolar capillary damage with disruption of alveolar membranes, interstitial and intra-alveolar extravasation of blood, and interstitial edema. The hemorrhage is most intense in the areas of lung abutting solid structures like ribs, liver, heart, vertebral column, and the costophrenic angles. As the lung edema progresses, alveoli fill with edema fluid, and alveolar ventilation and blood flow through the damaged lung diminish, causing impairment of gas exchange. Further discussion of the pathogenesis and pathophysiology of pulmonary edema is given in Chapter 6.

Clinical Signs

In mild pulmonary contusion, the patient may be slightly tachycardiac and tachypneic. He may complain of chest pain, but he is able to cough well. In the more severe cases of lung contusion, the patient is usually restless, tachypneic, and apprehensive. He coughs incessantly, but his cough is ineffective. Bronchial secretions are copious, and hemoptysis is frequently present.

Chest x ray abnormalities usually appear within an hour of injury; however, some patients have a lag time of 4–6 hr. Generally, two types of radiologic patterns are noted. The first is a patchy, poorly outlined density that may be localized or diffuse. The second, and less frequent, pattern is that of irregular, linear densities (infiltrates) with a peribronchial distribution. In addition, the contused lung may appear larger in size on the chest x ray, and the ipsilateral diaphragm may appear lower than the opposite side. Resolution of the chest x-ray abnormalities usually begins within 48–72 hr, but on occasion may take up to 14–21 days to completely clear. Slow resolution of the chest x-ray abnormalities suggests that complications, such as pneumonia or pulmonary embolus, have occurred.

As a rule, the clinical evaluation and initial chest x ray are not sensitive indicators of the degree of lung damage and the impairment of gas exchange. Therefore, arterial blood gas (ABG) measurements are mandatory. When present, hypoxemia must be promptly treated. An elevated Pa_{CO_2} in the presence of severe hypoxemia signifies severe contusion and carries a poor prognosis for the patient.

Treatment

The therapy of lung contusion depends on the extent of lung injury, as reflected by the impairment of gas exchange. In patients with mild lung contusion, the ABGs usually show a slight hypoxemia and possibly a mild hypocarbia. Therapy should consist of bed rest, judicious use of intravenous fluids, mild analgesia, pulmonary toilet, and supplemental oxygen to relieve the hypoxemia.

In the more severe cases of lung contusion, the arterial blood oxygen, Pa_{O_2}, is usually less than 70 mm Hg. There may also be a mild elevation of the Pa_{CO_2}. Therapy in these patients consists of endotracheal intubation and mechanical ventilation in an intensive care unit. The inspired oxygen concentration should be the lowest value that will maintain the patient's Pa_{O_2} above 55 mm Hg; positive end-expiratory pressure may be necessary to achieve this. Hemodynamic monitoring via a Swan–Ganz catheter and good tracheobronchial toilet are important. Although intravenous diuretics and albumin are frequently given, there is little proof of their efficacy in this setting. In general, intravenous fluids should be restricted to about 50 ml/hr. Methylprednisolone may also be given in a dose of 30 mg/kg initially, and then in divided doses for 3–4 days. Most of these patients will show clinical and radiographic improvement over 10–15 days; however, up to 15% of patients may die in spite of optimal therapy.

Finally, there is a small group of patients in whom the lung damage is so severe that even with ventilatory support adequate gas exchange is not possible. The only chance these patients have for survival is to be placed on an extracorporeal oxygenator in the hope that their lungs will eventually recover.

PULMONARY HEMATOMA

A pulmonary hematoma is the result of blood accumulating within the lung, in the space created by a pulmonary parenchymal disruption. It is an uncommon complication of blunt chest trauma, usually occurring in patients who sustain penetrating chest injuries with pulmonary lacerations (discussed in the next section).

The symptoms include chest pain, blood-streaked sputum, dyspnea, and a low-grade fever. In the absence of lung laceration, symptoms are rarely severe and usually subside in 7–10 days. The radiologic findings on the chest x ray include small, sharply defined, at times, spherical densities; irregularly shaped densities; and poorly defined, fuzzy infiltrates with radiolucencies. These densities usually reach their maximum opacification in 24 hr and disappear gradually over 1–3 weeks. Serious complications rarely develop without lung laceration, and therefore, therapy is usually symptomatic.

PULMONARY LACERATION

Pulmonary laceration is a rare complication of blunt chest trauma. Most commonly it is caused by bullet, knife, or shrapnel injuries that penetrate the chest wall. Fractured ribs or clavicles may also tear the lung. Lung laceration from blunt trauma without fractures is usually caused by a massive shock wave that disrupts the alveolar lining and visceral pleura causing a hemopneumothorax.

Clinical Signs

Symptoms (similar to those of lung contusion and hematoma) include chest pain and hemoptysis, which may be massive. The chest x ray is usually diagnostic, revealing a hemopneumothorax with a well-demarcated opacity in the lung substance that merges with the hemothorax.

Treatment

Therapy consists of immediate chest tube thoracostomy. Usually, two tubes are required, one placed anteriorly and superiorly to remove air, and the second placed in the dependent inferolateral position to remove blood. In most patients, when tube thoracostomy re-expands the lung, the air leak and bleeding promptly stop. However, persistent air leak and/ or bleeding requires early thoracotomy for repair and resection of the involved segment of lung. Chest tube drainage may be discontinued when drainage is less than 100 cc/24 hr, and there is no air leak.

PNEUMOMEDIASTINUM

Pneumomediastinum following blunt chest trauma results from rupture of either the tracheobronchial tree or the esophagus. Occasionally, compression of the chest wall against a closed glottis results in a sudden increase in alveolar pressure causing rupture of alveoli, escape of air into the pulmonary interstitial space, and dissection of the air along perivascular sheaths into the mediastinum, producing mediastinal emphysema. The complications of pneumomediastinum are listed in Table 3.

Fifty percent of patients have Hamman's sign, a systolic crunch heard over the heart and accentuated in the left lateral decubitus position. In addition, subcutaneous crepitation (air) is found in the tissues of the chest and neck. Chest x-ray findings include air along the cardiac silhouette and air in the subcutaneous tissues of the neck and anterior chest. All

TABLE 3. Complications of Pneumomediastinum

Pneumothorax	Subcutaneous emphysema in the neck
Pneumoprecordium	Subcutaneous emphysema of chest wall
Pneumopericardium	Compression of vena cava
Air in the retroperitoneal space	

patients with pneumomediastinum due to blunt chest trauma require a diagnostic assessment for tracheobronchial or esophageal rupture.

In most patients, the air in the subcutaneous tissues and in the mediastinum will resorb over a period of a few days, and no specific therapy is required. In a very rare case, cervical mediastinotomy or tracheostomy may be considered.

TRACHEOBRONCHIAL DISRUPTION

The true incidence of tracheobronchial disruption is difficult to establish since many people with such injuries die before reaching the hospital, and a smaller number of patients have a delayed onset of symptoms. Though uncommon, it is a serious and life-threatening injury with an overall mortality of approximately 30%. Any level of the trachea and major bronchi can be involved, although most injuries occur within 2.5 cm of the main carina. Lacerations of the bronchi and intrathoracic trachea are more common than those to the cervical trachea. The majority occur at the junction of the membranous and cartilaginous trachea. Vertical lacerations of the trachea occur posteriorly where there is no cartilaginous support. Most bronchial lacerations involve the mainstem bronchi and are usually transverse. They may be complete or incomplete and occur most frequently at the takeoff of the mainstem or upper-lobe bronchi, particularly on the right side. Bilateral bronchial rupture and rupture of lobar or segmental bronchi are uncommon.

Although the exact mechanism of tracheobronchial disruption is not known, three general theories exist. The trachea and/or bronchi can be

- Pulled apart when the chest is compressed and the lung is displaced laterally
- Actually blown apart, or ruptured, when the chest and lungs are compressed against a closed glottis
- Ripped apart by a shearing force generated by rapid deceleration of lung tissue during impact

Clinical Signs

The clinical presentation of intrathoracic tracheal or bronchial lacerations depends on whether there is a communication between the tear in the tracheobronchial tree and the pleura. When the ruptured airway communicates with the pleural space, a large pneumothorax with a persistent air leak occurs. Tension pneumothorax is uncommon, but subcutaneous and mediastinal emphysema may be present. Dyspnea, cyanosis, Hamman's sign, and variable degrees of hemoptysis can occur. Even when the bronchial transection is complete, the peribronchial tissues usually provide enough support to maintain an open airway and permit ventilation of the affected lung. As granulation tissue forms at the ends of the bronchus, 1–3 weeks after the injury, it can obstruct the airway, causing atelectasis. When the granulation tissue becomes epithelialized, a fibrous stricture develops. The obstructing stricture may result in a postobstructive pneumonitis and/or bronchiectasis with destruction of lung parenchyma.

There are no specific diagnostic radiologic findings of tracheobronchial disruption. However, Table 4 lists some of the important cues that suggest a rupture has occurred. If tracheobronchial disruption is suspected, bronchoscopy should be performed under operating room conditions with facilities ready for immediate thoracotomy. Occasionally, the laceration is not identified on the initial bronchoscopy, and a repeat bronchoscopy may be required.

Treatment

The treatment of choice is early surgical repair of the tracheobronchial disruption with bronchoscopy and dilatation of the anastomosis site at regular intervals. Treatment results are excellent in most patients when the repair is performed promptly. Occasionally, damage is so extensive that the entire lung must be resected. Ruptures of peripheral bronchi that have a persistent air leak, or cause atelectasis, usually require resection of the involved segment because the small diameter of the bronchus makes successful primary reanastomosis less likely.

TABLE 4. Radiologic Clues Suggesting Tracheobronchial Disruption

Pneumomediastinum	Fracture of any of the first five ribs
Deep cervical emphysema	Air density surrounding a bronchus
Pneumothorax	Obstruction in the course of an air-filled bronchus

CERVICAL TRACHEAL DISRUPTION

Typically, cervical tracheal disruption occurs in the setting of an automobile accident. The victim is sitting in the front seat; on impact, he strikes his head against the windshield and hyperextends his neck. This is called the "padded dashboard syndrome." In complete transection of the cervical trachea, the distal end of the trachea retracts into the mediastinum. If the flaccid pretracheal fascia remains intact, it may serve as a temporary airway. When the transection is incomplete and the pretracheal fascia remains intact, the patient may even be asymptomatic, from a respiratory standpoint, until a late stricture develops.

Clinical Signs

The diagnosis of cervical tracheal disruption must be considered in patients with blunt chest trauma who have respiratory distress and subcutaneous emphysema over the neck and anterior chest wall. Other clinical signs include

- Inspiratory stridor
- Hoarseness
- Localized tracheal pain or tenderness
- Hemoptysis
- Cyanosis

Complete tracheal transection usually presents as acute, severe, upper-airway obstruction.

Treatment

Bronchoscopy should be immediately performed to identify the site of injury. Because a rigid bronchoscope makes the diagnosis and establishes an airway at the same time, it is the instrument of choice, provided there are no other facial or neck injuries precluding its use. If the bronchoscope cannot be passed into the distal trachea, a tracheostomy should be performed immediately to establish an airway. When the patient is stable, surgical repair of the trachea should be undertaken without delay. At the time of tracheal repair, the esophagus must be carefully examined and repaired if lacerated.

ESOPHAGEAL RUPTURE

Esophageal rupture is an uncommon complication of blunt chest trauma. However, if undetected it causes severe acute mediastinitis.

The presenting signs of traumatic esophageal rupture may include

- Dyspnea
- Cyanosis
- Upper-abdominal pain
- Elevated blood pressure
- Subcutaneous emphysema in the neck and anterior chest

The chest x ray can show

- Pneumothorax
- Hydropneumothorax
- Subcutaneous and mediastinal emphysema

The diagnosis is confirmed by an esophagogram, but may occasionally require a careful esophagoscopy (when the esophagogram is not diagnostic). Lacerations are usually linear and, although they can occur in any portion of the esophagus, are most frequently found in the distal one-third. Therapy of a ruptured esophagus consists of early diagnosis and prompt surgical repair.

CHYLOTHORAX

Chylothorax, an extremely rare complication of blunt chest trauma, is caused by disruption of the thoracic duct above the level of the diaphragm. Two or ten days after injury to the thoracic duct, chyle appears in the pleural space; however, symptoms of respiratory compromise occur only after large amounts of chyle have accumulated. The diagnosis is made by obtaining milky, white pleural fluid at thoracentesis. Since chyle appears to be bacteriostatic, infection rarely develops in chylothorax. Therapy consists of either repeated thoracenteses or closed-tube thoracostomy and attempts to reduce chyle formation by decreasing oral intake through parenteral hyperalimentation. When the production of chylous fluid begins to decrease, the patient is fed an oral diet devoid of long-chain triglycerides and fatty acids. The fat content of the diet can be supplemented with medium-chain triglycerides. If the fluid accumulation persists, thoracotomy with ligation of the thoracic duct, or ducts, at their entry into the chest, just above the diaphragm, and pleurodesis are usually necessary.

RUPTURE OF THE DIAPHRAGM

Although traumatic rupture of the diaphragm may occur with blunt chest trauma, it is more frequently seen in abdominal trauma. Most cases of diaphragmatic rupture are the result of trauma sustained in an automobile accident. Less common causes include falls from great height, animal kicks, and crushing injuries.

Often diaphragmatic rupture is diagnosed long after the traumatic event; therefore, its true incidence is unknown. The left diaphragm is more commonly ruptured than the right. Usually, the tear in the diaphragm is radial and occurs on the posterolateral aspect. The laceration is frequently large enough to permit herniation of abdominal viscera such as stomach, colon, small bowel, spleen, and omentum. Because the force required to rupture the diaphragm is large, there is a high incidence of associated injuries, including multiple rib and skeletal fractures, ruptured spleen and/or liver, perforation of the colon or small bowel, and pancreatic injury. Rupture of the right diaphragm is associated with a higher incidence of multiple injuries compared to the left.

Left Diaphragm

One-third of patients with left diaphragmatic ruptures have small tears and no symptoms. Usually, there is associated left-upper-quadrant abdominal pain, left-lower-chest pain, and referred left-shoulder pain. Massive herniation of abdominal viscera may cause mediastinal shift, respiratory distress, hypotension, and cyanosis. Physical examination may reveal a scaphoid abdomen with bowel sounds in the chest.

The x-ray findings associated with left diaphragmatic rupture are listed in Table 5. The diagnosis is confirmed by inserting a nasogastric tube into the stomach prior to obtaining a chest x ray and/or by a Gastrografin upper gastrointestinal study. Some patients may require a barium enema to identify herniated colon in the chest.

TABLE 5. X-Ray Findings in Traumatic Left Diaphragmatic Rupture

---

"Apparently elevated" left hemidiaphragm
Obscured or irregularly elevated left hemidiaphragm
An unusual gas density, or bubble, above the left hemidiaphragm
Atelectasis, usually platelike, adjacent to elevated left hemidiaphragm
Pleural effusion
An air–fluid level (or multiple air–fluid levels) in the left chest
Mediastinal shift to the right

The treatment of acute left diaphragmatic rupture is surgical repair of the diaphragm through a left thoracotomy incision; some patients may also require a laparotomy when the extent of injury is great.

Right Diaphragm

The clinical symptoms and physical findings of right-diaphragmatic rupture are similar to those described above. The x-ray appearance depends on the degree of herniation of the liver through the diaphragm. In some patients the entire liver is herniated into the right chest and looks like an elevated diaphragm. In other patients only a portion of the liver is herniated, and there is a "mushroom" appearance to the dome of the right diaphragm. Occasionally, the entire liver and colon can be seen in the right chest. Currently the best procedure for confirmation of rupture of the right diaphragm involves the combined use of liver and lung scans. The treatment of right-diaphragmatic rupture consists of stabilization of the patient's acute injuries followed by prompt surgical repair through a right thoracotomy; occasionally, a combined laparotomy is also required depending on the size of the herniation.

BIBLIOGRAPHY

1. Daughtry DC: *Thoracic Trauma*. Boston, Little, Brown, 1980.
2. Douglass AM, Paul ME, Finley RJ, et al: Chest trauma—Current morbidity and mortality. *J Trauma* 17:547–553, 1977.
3. Kirsch MM, Sloan H: *Blunt Chest Trauma. General Principles of Management*. Boston, Little, Brown, 1977.
4. Ratcliff JL, Fletcher JR, Kopriou CJ, et al: Pulmonary contusion, a management problem. *J Thorac Cardiovasc Surg* 62:638–644, 1971.
5. Sankaran S, Wilson RF: Factors affecting prognosis in patients with flail chest. *J Thorac Cardiovasc Surg* 60:402–410, 1970.
6. Wilson RF, Murray C, Antonenko DR: Non-penetrating thoracic injuries. *Surg Clin North Am* 57:17–36, 1977.

CHAPTER 9

Upper-Airway Emergencies

Kenneth Dickie

CLINICAL SIGNS AND SYMPTOMS

Acute upper-airway emergencies develop from mechanical obstruction of the airway which, if not reversed, leads to asphyxiation. The signs and symptoms of the obstruction are relative to the amount of the obstruction and the speed at which it occurs. Obstruction is caused by a wide variety of disorders, which have in common a local mechanical effect causing the symptoms of obstruction, but may, in addition, have other systemic effects that are more specific for the diagnosis.

The signs of obstruction are affected by the level of consciousness. The conscious patient will usually exhibit anxiety, gagging, salivation, lack of phonation, poor air movement, and possibly cyanosis. The unconscious patient will exhibit intercostal indrawing, accessory respiratory muscle activity, and lack of air movement at the nose and mouth (see Fig. 1).

In general, the patient with acute airway obstruction presents with

- Sudden shortness of breath
- Difficulty moving air
- Sensation of obstruction to air movement in the neck
- Difficulty speaking
- Stridor (high-pitched, continuous sound)
- Anxiety
- Gagging
- Salivation
- Cyanosis

Kenneth Dickie • Division of Pulmonary Diseases and Allergy, George Washington University School of Medicine and Health Sciences, Washington, D.C. 20037; Veterans Administration Medical Center, Washington, D.C. 20422.

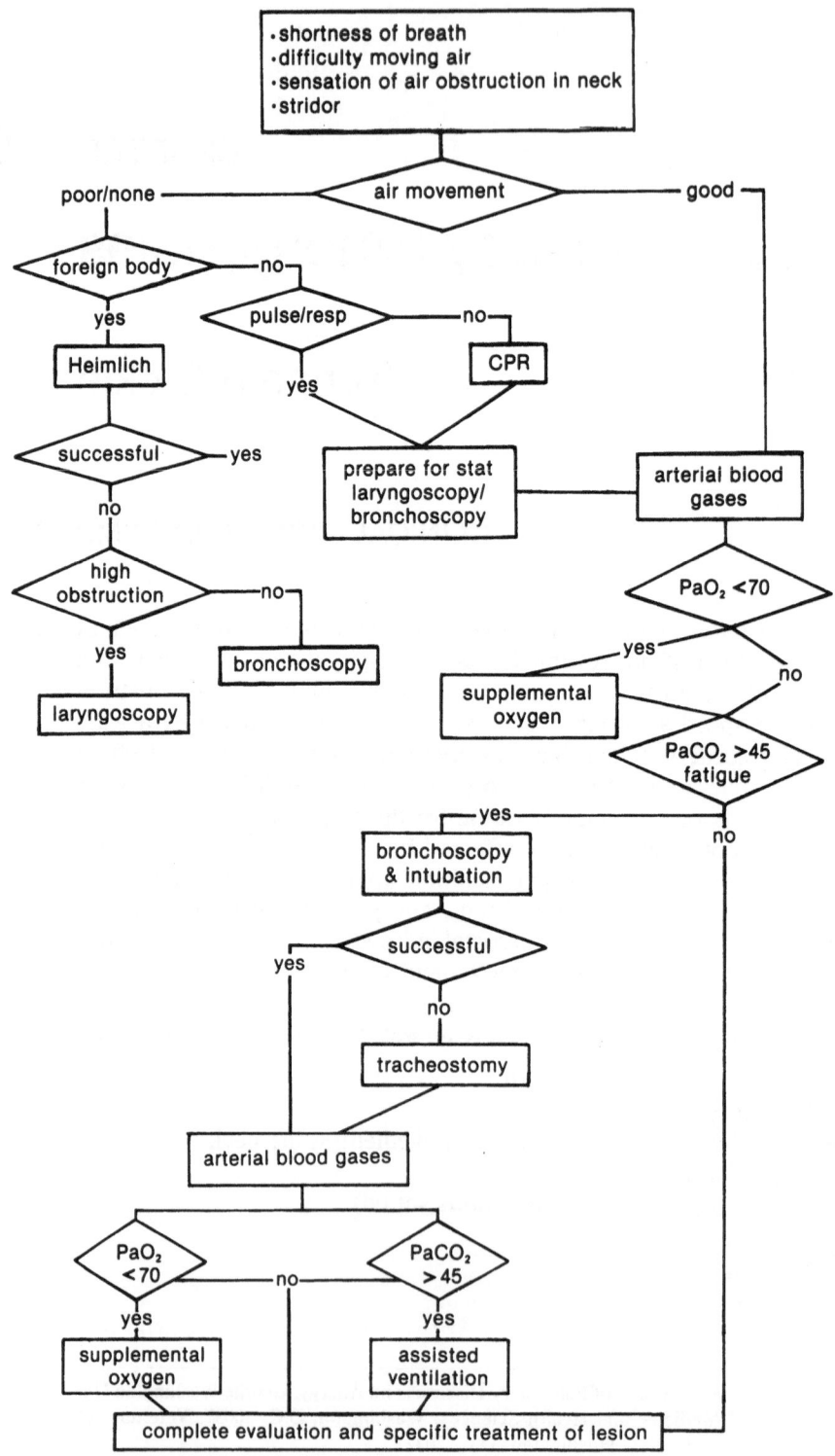

FIGURE 1. Algorithm for emergency evaluation and management of acute upper-airway obstruction.

Incomplete obstruction presents a variable combination of gagging, coughing, wheezing, dyspnea, hoarseness, and stridor. With complete obstruction, the patient cannot breath or talk, will clutch the neck between thumb and forefinger, and appears in acute anxiety needing assistance.

Local signs and symptoms may assist in determiniing a specific cause or location of the obstructing lesion. Local swelling from tumor or infection results in displacement and dysfunction of normal tissue. Pain, tenderness, and redness may be seen with infections. Look for dysphagia, suprasternal and supraclavicular retraction, trismus, elevation of the tongue, pain on moving the hyoid, and swelling in the submandibular and neck regions. Lacerations, abrasions, or scars may be present from surgery or trauma.

DIFFERENTIAL DIAGNOSIS

Airway obstruction in the adult may be caused by a great variety of unrelated, rare, and uncommon disorders (Table 1). These disorders share the common potential problem of obstructing the airway. The obstruction must be recognized when it occurs and may, as a lifesaving measure, require emergency measures to bypass the obstruction. Once the acute obstruction has been diagnosed and treated, the investigation of the specific etiology of the obstructing lesion, if not determined during the emergency care, can proceed. As can be seen from Table 1, the range of investigation could be extensive, but is not an emergency and will not be discussed here.

Aspiration of food during meals is the most frequent cause of upper-airway obstruction requiring emergency treatment. It is frequently ac-

TABLE 1. Disorders associated with Upper-Airway Obstruction

Trauma	Cysts or neoplasms
Accidents involving the upper-airway region	Of the larynx and trachea
Endotracheal intubation	Vocal cord paralysis
Tracheostomy	Infections
Irritation from bronchoscopy	Laryngotracheobronchitis
Penetrating neck wounds (stabbing or gunshot)	Acute supraglottitis (epiglottitis)
Airway burn	Acute adenotonsillitis
Foreign body aspiration	Diphtheria
Aspiration or inhalation of irritants and corrosives	Sleep apnea syndromes
Congenital abnormalities	Tracheobronchiomegaly (Ehlers–Danlos syndrome)
Involving the oropharynx, larynx, trachea, or jaw	Tracheomalacia
Laryngeal dysfunction	Hypothyroidism with goiter
	Hereditary angioedema
	Allergies and anaphylaxis

companied by the imbibing of alcohol prior to and/or in association with the meal and requires immediate therapy, instituted by nearby observers. As a result, this problem is frequently fully, or partially, resolved prior to being seen by medical practitioners, but it may require further medical attention to remove aspirated material.

INVESTIGATING THE OBSTRUCTION

Obstruction may be due to an abnormality inside the airway, to a lesion of the airway itself, or to compression from disease outside the airway. The common effect is to reduce the cross-sectional area of the airway, reducing the airflow to and from the lungs. Clinical evaluation is needed to determine the urgency of therapy; the location and extent of obstruction; the type of obstruction, intrinsic or extrinsic; its pathologic cause; and the means of therapy.

Immediate Assessment

Upper-airway obstructions are potentially life-threatening emergencies. Therefore, prior to proceeding with an extensive history and evaluation, determine the urgency of treatment from

- A past breathing problem
- The progression of the dyspnea
- The amount of respiratory distress
- Examination of the throat and neck
- Examination of the chest
- Arterial blood gases and pH

If the time course, progression, and severity of the dyspnea suggest impending respiratory failure, that is:

- Rapid progression of dyspnea in minutes or hours
- Poor respirations and breath sounds
- Cyanosis, weakness, lethargy, disorientation, or coma
- Elevated arterial P_{CO_2}

prepare for endotracheal intubation, and possible tracheostomy. In this emergency situation, failed attempts at intubation may result in immediate and serious respiratory failure and possibly death. Therefore, use the best location and the most highly skilled and experienced staff that is available for the procedure. While it is imperative to prepare for and sometimes perform an emergency procedure, whenever possible, delay the intubation or tracheostomy until the lesion and its location have been identified and preparation has been made for the procedure. Intubation under controlled conditions using bronchoscopic guidance, or tracheostomy after adequate preparation, will avoid many potential errors.

History

The history will provide information about the severity of the lesion, its progression, the need for immediate intervention, and the likelihood of congenital diseases, infections, complications of long-standing lung diseases, trauma, sleep apnea, and other disorders listed in Table 1.

Physical Examination

Inspection of the head, neck, and chest will provide further data with which to estimate the severity of the obstruction, the urgency of treatment, and indication of the likely pathology. Trauma or scars from surgery, swelling and redness from infections, gross obesity with snorting respiration, obvious somnolence association with obstructive sleep apnea, and congenital abnormalities may be seen. Inspection of the breathing pattern can be used to separate patients requiring no intervention from patients with strong respiratory movement but requiring an endotracheal tube or tracheostomy and from other patients with weakening or weak respiration requiring both intubation and mechanical ventilatory support. Thick, fat, short necks may need long-term endotracheal tubes rather than a tracheostomy. High, occluding lesions may indicate immediate tracheostomy.

Endoscopy

Although the cause, extent, location, and treatment of the obstructing lesion may be apparent by history and external inspection, most often endoscopy will be needed. Lesions that are high in the airway may be seen by direct or indirect laryngoscopy, but lower obstructions will need bronchoscopy. During these examinations, the airway is assessed for patency of the lumen, the condition of the mucosa, the integrity of the bronchial walls, the presence of intrinsic lesions, and evidence of external compression. Washings, brushings, and/or biopsies of abnormalities will assist in identifying neoplasms. Cultures are used to specify the infecting organisms and their antibiotic sensitivities. During bronchoscopy, the partially occluded airway may be totally occluded, thereby precipitating an acute emergency. This usually can be avoided by experienced personnel, exercising care in inserting and manipulating the bronchoscope, but a complete examination may not be possible because of the narrowed airway lumen.

Arterial Blood pH and Gases

Blood gases are the quickest and best clinical measure of overall respiratory function. Frequent measurements are needed to monitor the respiratory status of the severely ill patient. Acidosis indicates actual, or potential, respiratory insufficiency. An elevated Pa_{CO_2}, means hypoventilation, either due to the incapacity to move sufficient air past a major obstruction or from fatigue caused by the increased work of breathing through the obstructed airway. Hyperventilation, indicated by a low Pa_{CO_2}, may be seen initially. As the patient improves, the carbon dioxide will increase into the normal range. The improving patient will look and feel better, with less respiratory distress and more responsiveness to the surroundings. Occasionally a diagnostic error may occur when a patient who appears more comfortable, with less distress and dyspnea, and may be going to sleep is, instead of improving, developing acute respiratory failure and about to stop breathing altogether. If doubt exists, arterial blood gas analysis will distinguish between normalization and respiratory failure. With respiratory failure, the pH becomes acid and the Pa_{CO_2} will rise above normal.

X Rays

X rays of the neck, posteroanterior and lateral, may show the narrowing of the airway and some indication of the state of the surrounding soft tissue. A true lateral exposure is best for assessing the upper airways. A computerized tomography (CT) scan gives a more accurate visualization of the airway and the obstructing lesion. When bronchoscopy is not a realistic option, or the examination cannot be satisfactorily completed, the CT scan is useful to assess the state of the airway dimensions and the surrounding tissue.

Pulmonary Function

An indication of the level and severity of the obstruction can be assessed from the inspired and expired flow–volume measurements. A fixed obstruction will reduce both inspired and expired flow with a "flattening'' (plateau) of the loop. Variable extrathoracic lesions will reduce and flatten the inspiratory tracing. Variable intrathoracic lesions reduce and flatten the expiratory recording.

MANAGEMENT

The objective of emergency therapy is to improve the ventilation of the lungs by reducing the obstruction to airflow and, when necessary, by providing mechanical ventilation and supplemental oxygen (Fig. 1).

Assess the Need for Intervention

The amount of obstruction that is present and the likelihood of progression to further obstruction are determined from the history of the onset of the obstructive symptoms, the duration and progression of the respiratory symptoms, the current dyspnea, and observation of the work of breathing. A rapid onset of symptoms with severe, increasing dyspnea indicates, in conjunction with objective findings of obstruction and respiratory failure, an urgent need to reduce the obstruction by intubation or tracheostomy. The physical examination will produce evidence of mechanical obstruction such as wheezes, stridor, or snorting respiration and, sometimes, lesions in the head, neck, or upper chest that are causing obstruction.

Arterial blood gases are used to determine the presence or absence of respiratory failure. Serial measurements will show subsequent progression to normal or to respiratory failure. The presence of respiratory failure requires reducing the obstruction and often will require mechanical ventilatory assistance.

Pulmonary function tests will show overall ventilatory capacity and discriminate between intra- and extrathoracic, variable or fixed obstructions, but treatment will generally require more specific information than can be gained from these tests.

Assess the Location and Extent of the Obstruction

This requires laryngoscopic or bronchoscopic examination, supplemented by roentgenograms and/or axial tomography. As mentioned previously, a pulmonary flow–volume loop may supplement these tests.

Ensure a Patent Airway

Without evidence of respiratory failure, no emergency treatment is necessary. Observe the patient for evidence of tiring or progression toward respiratory failure, which would require emergency treatment. Meanwhile, proceed with the investigation of the obstruction.

If respiratory failure is present or imminent, and the airway is sufficiently patent to allow safe passage of a tube, insert an oral or nasal endotracheal tube. The endotracheal tube may be inserted over a bronchoscope to ease the passage and decrease the trauma of entry. In general, the endotracheal tube is used for lesions that are considered reversible and is used as a temporary airway support. With experience in maintaining the indwelling tube and improved design of tubes, the "temporary" period that is considered safe and effective has gradually increased to several weeks.

A tracheostomy will be necessary

- For lesions that are permanent
- For lesions that cause nearly complete obstruction that prevents insertion of an endotracheal tube
- For airways having a fragile surface that will be seriously eroded by passage of an endotracheal tube, resulting in serious damage or bleeding in the airway or surrounding tissue

When possible, the tracheotomy can follow an emergency endotracheal intubation; the tracheotomy is then done under improved, better controlled operating procedure, after the condition of the patient has stabilized and a complete assessment of the needs of the patient has been made.

Bronchoscopically guided laser therapy is used to open an airway channel for obstructing lesions, usually tumors, that occlude much of the distal tracheal lumen within the chest and cannot be bypassed by either an endotracheal tube or a tracheostomy.

Determine the Etiology of the Obstructing Lesion

After the emergency situation has been controlled, a full investigation of the cause and treatment of the obstruction is undertaken. Frequently, the specific etiology of the obstructing lesion will have been determined by the biopsies, washings, and/or brushings during the emergency bronchoscopy.

Treatment

Treatment, other than establishing a patent airway, varies with the etiology and is specific for each disease rather than for the airway component of the disease. One problem, the aspiration of foreign bodies, is unique to the airway, and the treatment is outlined here.

Foreign bodies are usually gagged or coughed up prior to reaching medical attention. The patient can assist the expulsion of the foreign body by coughing while placing the upper airway in a dependent position by lying over a chair, or bed, with the head down. Foreign bodies that are not spontaneously removed by the patient's own efforts can be removed by one of several methods.

Insert the forefinger along the inside of the patient's cheek, sweeping the finger back along the cheek to the pharynx, across the pharynx to the inside of the other cheek, and then forward along the inside of the other cheek. This maneuver may remove the foreign body even when the object is not touched by the finger.

Deliver three sharp knocks between the shoulder blades with the side of the lightly closed fist. This is reportedly successful, but may, occasionally, result in further lodging of the foreign body rather than its dislodgment.

A third method, known as the Heimlich maneuver, is to stand behind the patient and, while having the patient bend forward slightly at the waist, allowing the head, arms, and torso to hang forward, to wrap both arms around the patient with one forearm across the upper abdomen (below the ribs), grasp the wrist that is around the patient with the other hand, and rapidly, but firmly squeeze the upper abdomen. This causes a rapid exhalation, which dislodges the foreign body. Similar compression of the subdiaphragmatic abdomen can be used with the victim in other positions.

Failure of these three maneuvers requires removal of the obstruction by instrumentation or bypass of the obstruction by tracheostomy. Occasionally, a large-caliber hypodermic needle inserted into the trachea, through the cricothyroid membrane below the obstruction, may serve as a temporary airway.

BIBLIOGRAPHY

1. Arabian A, Spagnolo SV: Laser therapy in lung cancer. *Chest* 86:519–523, 1984.
2. Boster SR, Martinez SA: Acute upper airway obstruction in the adult. 1. Causative disease processes. Postgrad Med 72:50–52, 55–57, 1982.
3. Boster SR, Martinez SA: Acute upper airway obstruction in the adult. 2. Causative events. Postgrad Med 72:61–63, 66–67, 1982.   ·
4. Bristow G: Acute upper airway obstruction. *Semin Respir Med* 2:1–4, 1980.
5. Heimlich HJ: Pop goes the cafe coronary. Emergency Med 6:154–155, 1974.
6. McCullough D: Surgical management of acute upper airway obstruction. *Semin Respir Med* 2:6–11, 1980.

PART III

Chronic Lung Disease with Acute Respiratory Decompensation

CHAPTER 10

Acute Respiratory Failure in the Patient with Chronic Airflow Obstruction

Samuel V. Spagnolo

Respiratory failure occurs when gas exchange is impaired. Mild degrees of respiratory failure with hypoxemia or hypercarbia may be present for many years without apparent serious physiologic consequences because of the body's normal compensatory mechanisms. The severity of respiratory failure and the need for urgent therapeutic intervention depend on the rate and degree of deterioration in gas exchange as reflected in the arterial blood gases (ABG). Life-threatening, acute respiratory failure occurs when gas exchange is deteriorating rapidly, with accelerated alterations in acid–base chemistry. Abrupt alterations in gas exchange (occurring over minutes to several days) that lower the Pa_{O_2} below 55 mm Hg or lower the pH below 7.30 (by raising the Pa_{CO_2} above 50 mm Hg) require rapid and aggressive therapy.

This chapter focuses on acute, life-threatening respiratory failure occurring in patients with underlying severe, chronic airflow obstruction (CAO), primarily caused by *emphysema* and *chronic bronchitis*, who previously functioned in a compensated state of chronic respiratory insufficiency.

PRECIPITATING EVENTS AND PATHOPHYSIOLOGY

A variety of medical and/or surgical insults can precipitate acute respiratory failure in patients with chronic pulmonary insufficiency. Often

Samuel V. Spagnolo • Division of Pulmonary Diseases and Allergy, Department of Medicine, George Washington University School of Medicine and Health Sciences, Washington, D.C. 20037; Pulmonary Disease Section, Veterans Administration Medical Center, Washington, D.C. 20422.

TABLE 1. Factors Commonly Precipitating Acute
Decompensation in Patients with Chronic Airflow Obstruction

Viral or bacterial bronchitis	Pulmonary emboli
Viral or bacterial pneumonia	Pleural effusion
Spontaneous pneumothorax	General anesthesia
Left-heart failure	Sedative drugs
Abdominal or thoracic surgery	Poor compliance with prescribed medications

a viral or bacterial infection leads to increased airflow obstruction. With such infections, bronchial mucus is secreted into the airways at a faster rate than it can be cleared; in addition, there is frequently an increase in spasm of bronchial smooth muscle. Additional factors precipitating acute respiratory failure are listed in Table 1. As a consequence of any of these events, ventilation–perfusion ratios ($\dot{V}/\dot{Q}$) are further altered throughout the lung, causing increased arterial hypoxemia and hypercarbia. The degree of hypercarbia and hypoxemia is determined by the severity of the increased airway resistance and the ability of the lung's compensatory mechanisms to match ventilation (airflow) with perfusion (blood flow). The patient's initial compensatory response to the worsening of pulmonary gas exchange is an increase in respiratory rate; the elevated respiratory rate is an attempt to raise minute ventilation. In addition, the actual muscular work of breathing increases because the pump (lung) works against higher resistance. These compensatory ventilatory responses can be blunted because

- The respiratory muscle work required to overcome the high airway resistance and maintain adequate ventilation is too great for the patient to sustain.
- Some patients with CAO have abnormal central and peripheral respiratory chemoreceptor responses; consequently, a falling Pa_{O_2} and rising Pa_{CO_2} may stimulate less central ventilatory activity (output).

In addition, to these airflow and central respiratory drive problems, chronic and acute *alveolar* hypoxia causes constriction of pulmonary arterioles. As a result, pulmonary vascular resistance rises and right-heart failure (cor pulmonale) can occur suddenly.

Although patients with a chronically reduced Pa_{O_2} appear to tolerate acutely lowered levels of Pa_{O_2} better than normal people, these levels cannot be tolerated for long and eventually lead to tissue and cell death. When the Pa_{O_2} persists below 30 mm Hg, irreversible brain and myocardial damage occurs.

CLINICAL FINDINGS AND DIAGNOSIS

Patients with CAO often exhibit the following symptoms and signs:

- Chronic daily cough
- Chronic dyspnea
- Chest tightness
- Wheezing
- Daily sputum production

When acute decompensation of respiratory function occurs in these patients, they usually complain of

- Increasing shortness of breath and wheezing
- Increasing difficulty in raising sputum
- Change in sputum color from white to yellow or green

If the patient is cyanotic or unresponsive, an obvious life-threatening emergency is present. In this situation, CO_2 narcosis and severe hypoxemia (unless the patient is receiving supplemental oxygen) are present. Findings on the physical examination that suggest hypoxic hypercarbia include

- Hypertension
- Focal neurologic signs
- Miosis
- Papilledema
- Diminished or absent breath sounds

Immediate analysis of ABG is mandatory to confirm the diagnosis of severe impairment of respiratory gas exchange.

TREATMENT

Two basic physiologic principles are involved in the therapy of patients with acute, life-threatening respiratory failure and CAO.

- Improve Pa_{O_2} and tissue oxygenation by
  - Utilizing controlled low-flow oxygen therapy
- Improve lung $\dot{V}/\dot{Q}$ by
  - Clearing the airways of secretions
  - Relieving bronchospasm and inflammation
  - Treating infection (and/or colonization)
  - Reducing pulmonary vascular resistance
  - Improving cardiac output

Specific measures to fulfill these objectives are described below; Fig. 1 summarizes the emergency management.

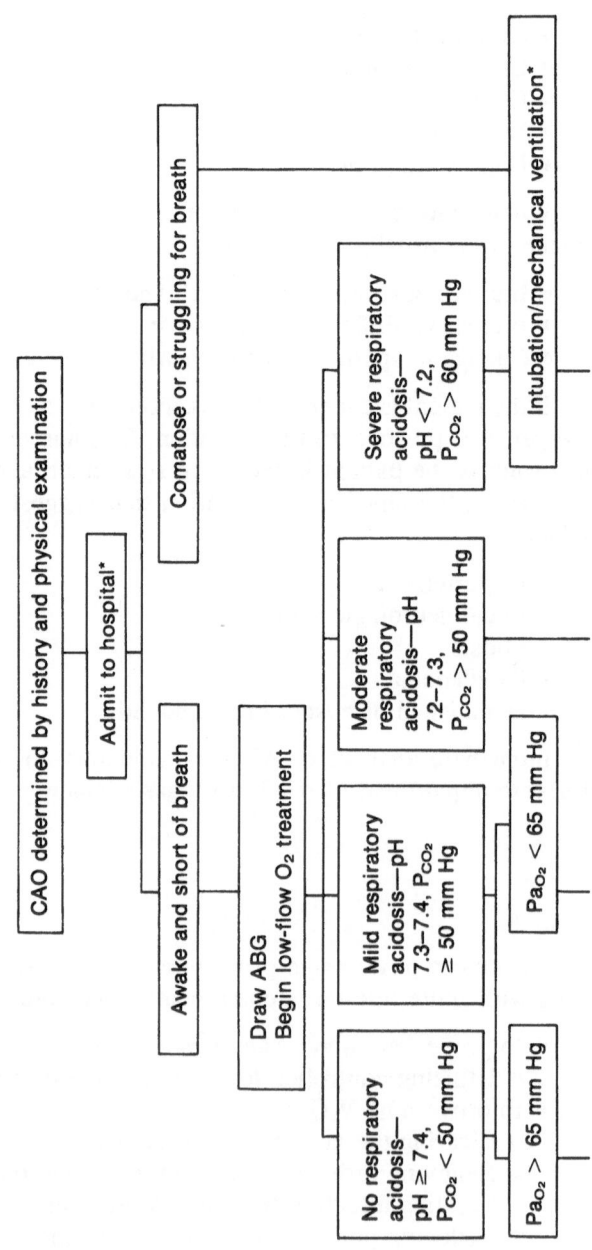

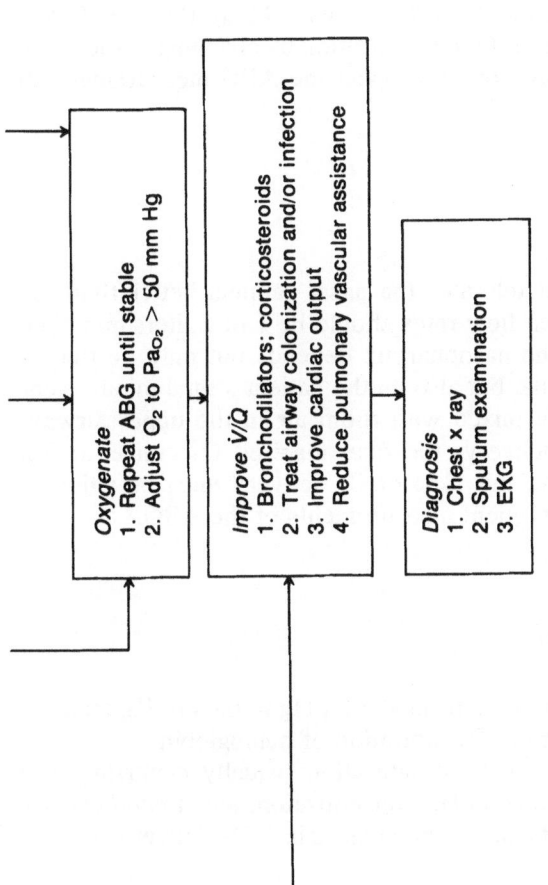

FIGURE 1. Emergency management of acute respiratory failure in chronic airflow obstruction (CAO). *, See text for explanation.

LOW-FLOW CONTROLLED OXYGEN THERAPY

Masks (Venturi-Type)

Venturi masks mix oxygen and room air at fixed ratios and deliver oxygen (O_2) concentrations at one of the following concentrations; 24, 26, 28, 31, 35, or 40%. When first initiating therapy in these patients, choose a mask that delivers 24 or 28% O_2. The adequacy of this O_2 concentration should be assessed 20–30 min after initiating therapy by repeating the measurement of the ABG. If the desired Pa_{O_2} ($Pa_{O_2} > 50$) has not been achieved, increase the O_2 concentration by changing to the mask of the next highest concentration and repeat the ABG measurement 20 min later.

Nasal Cannula

Frequently, the patient tolerates the nasal cannula better than the Venturi mask. Initial oxygen flow rates should be 1 or 2 liters/min. The final O_2 concentration in the nasopharynx depends not only on the O_2 flow rate through the cannula, but also on the patient's total minute ventilation because the oxygen mixed with room air in the upper airway. With this method of O_2 delivery, the final inspired O_2 concentration (FI_{O_2}) is variable; therefore, this type of O_2 delivery *must* be adjusted according to results of subsequent measurements of the ABG.

Notes about Oxygen Therapy

- Small increases in the Pa_{O_2} from 40 mm Hg to 60 mm Hg result in a marked increase in the O_2 saturation of hemoglobin.
- With (90%) hemoglobin (Hb) saturation (usually occurring at a Pa_{O_2} of 60 mm Hg), a good Hb concentration, and a *good* cardiac output, these patients should have sufficient O_2 delivery to meet metabolic needs.
- Often, after supplemental controlled O_2 is given to these patients, a slight amount of ventilatory drive is lost and a small (3–5 mm Hg) rise in Pa_{CO_2} occurs. This small increase is *not* an indication to discontinue or reduce the supplemental O_2, but does require additional ABG measurements to determine that further hypercapnea is not developing.
- Supplemental controlled O_2 therapy should not be discontinued until the patient can maintain an adequate Pa_{O_2} on room air.

- Controlled oxygen therapy by nasal cannula is effective in patients who are mouth breathers.
- Abrupt removal of all supplemental O_2 from a patient with severe hypercapnea ($Pa_{CO_2} > 65$ mm Hg) and a large (>30 mm Hg) alveolar–arterial O_2 gradient may result in rapid reduction of the Pa_{O_2} to a level that could be fatal.

IMPROVING LUNG $\dot{V}/\dot{Q}$

Clearing Airway Secretions

Inspissated secretions are best expelled by

- Effective coughing
- Careful nasotracheal suctioning
- Chest physiotherapy

Relieving Bronchospasm and Reducing Inflammation

Bronchodilators are given to lower airway resistance. Either parenteral aminophylline (see Table 2) or a nebulized (or parenteral) adrenergic agonist (see Table 3) may be used. Even when wheezing is not heard, bronchodilators may be helpful to these patients for the following reasons:

- Patients with acute, severe bronchospasm may have little or absent wheezing because of reduced airflow.

TABLE 2. Intravenous Aminophylline Therapy[a]

	Yes	No
A. Loading dose		
1. Has the patient been taking maintenance aminophylline as an outpatient?	3 mg/kg	6 mg/kg
2. Does the patient have evidence of a ventricular arrhythmia?	3 mg/kg	6 mg/kg
B. Maintenance dose		
1. Does the patient have heart or liver disease?	0.3 mg/kg per hour	0.6 mg/kg per hour
2. Does the patient have evidence of a ventricular arrththmia?	0.3 mg/kg per hour	0.6 mg/kg per hour

[a] These are suggested doses, and final doses should be adjusted on the basis of theophylline blood levels.

TABLE 3. Comparison of Sympathomimetic Bronchodilators[a]

	Albuterol	Terbutaline	Metaproterenol	Bitolterol	Isoetharine	Isoproterenol	Epinephrine
Metered aerosols							
Mg per puff	0.09 mg	0.2 mg	0.65 mg	0.37 mg	0.34 mg	0.125 mg	0.2 mg
Puffs per use	1–2	1–2	2–3	2–3	1–2	1–2	1–2
Frequency of use	q 4–6 hr	q 4–6 hr	q 3–6 hr	q 6–8 hr	q 3–4 hr	q 3–6 hr[b]	q 4–6 hr[b]
Solutions for nebulization							
Concentration	Not available	Not available	5%	Not available	1%	1:200 (0.5%)	1.25% or 2.25%
Volume of solution			0.2–0.3 ml		0.25–0.5 ml	0.3–0.5 ml	2–3 ml
Volume of saline diluent			2–3 ml		2–3 ml	2–3 ml	None
Frequency of use			q 4–6 hr		q 4–6 hr	q 2–4 hr[b]	2–3 inhalations q 15–30 min[b]
Subcutaneous							
Concentration	Not available	1 mg/ml	Not available	Not available	Not available	Not available	1:1000 (aqueous)
Dose per use		0.25–0.5 mg					0.3–0.5 ml
Frequency of use		q 4–6 hr					q 30 min 1:200 (aqueous suspension) 0.1–0.3 ml q 6 hr

[a] Adult recommendations only.
[b] Routine use not recommended.

- Small changes in airway resistance can significantly improve airflow, ventilation, and consequently gas exchange.
- Theophylline acts as a central respiratory stimulant.
- Theophylline will improve contractility of the diaphragm and delay the onset of diaphragmatic fatigue.

Methylprednisolone intravenously (0.5 mg/kg every 6 hr for 72 hr) will improve the FEV_1 during the first 72 hr of hospitalization in some patients. The exact mechanism of action is not known, but the drug is believed to reduce local airway edema. In individuals showing a response to initial steroid administration, treatment may be continued with alternate-day prednisone therapy for several weeks.

Treating Infection and/or Bacterial Colonization of the Lower Airways

Antibiotics appear helpful in those seriously ill CAO patients with heavy sputum production. Many patients with CAO and mucus hypersecretion already have bacterial (*Hemophilus influenzae; Streptococcus pneumoniae*) colonization in the lower respiratory tract. Further disruption of airway defense mechanisms may permit these bacteria or other microbes (*Mycoplasma pneumonia, Chlamydia,* anaerobic bacteria, and other gram-negative bacteria) newly introduced into the lower airway to invade tissues, causing overt clinical disease.

Choice of Antimicrobial Agent(s)

In general, the antimicrobial agent(s) used in the acutely decompensated patient will depend on whether acute bronchitis and/or overt clinical pneumonia is present. The diagnosis and treatment of acute, life-threatening pneumonia is fully described in Chapter 4.

For the patient with *only* acute or worsening chronic bronchitis, the antimicrobial agent or agents chosen for treatment should be effective against the bacteria identified by gram stain of a lower-respiratory-tract specimen (sputum). Bacteria found most often by gram stain in this setting include *S. pneumoniae, H.* influenzae, and *Branhamella catarrhalis* (formerly *Neisseria catarrhalis*). Antimicrobial agents useful for the treatment of these bacteria include the following:

- Penicillin G
- Erythromycin
- Amoxicillin/potassium clavulanate
- Sulfamethoxazole—trimethoprim
- Cephalosporins (cephalexin, cefaclor, cefotaxime, ceftazidime)

It is unusual for the Gram stain of the sputum to reveal only Gram-negative, uniform-appearing bacteria. When this occurs, therapy with third- or fourth-generation cephalosporins, such as cefotaxime or ceftazidime, should be initiated until identification of the specific bacteria is available from examination of bacterial cultures.

If the Gram stain of sputum in these patients reveals only polymorphonuclear white blood cells and *no* visible bacteria (and the patient does not have pneumonia), then empiric antimicrobial therapy with a tetracycline (doxycycline) or erythromycin can be used until further evaluation has been completed.

Reducing Pulmonary Vascular Resistance

The correction of alveolar hypoxemia with administration of supplemental O_2 is usually effective in lowering acute elevations in pulmonary artery pressure (PAP). Vasodilator drugs such as the calcium channel blocker nifedipine may reduce PAP; they should be used only with ongoing monitoring of the PAP.

Improving Cardiac Output

Occasionally, right and left ventricular failure are prominent features in severely decompensated respiratory patients. Identifying left-heart failure in this situation often requires measure of the pulmonary capillary wedge pressure. In the absence of left-heart failure, failure of the right ventricle is usually due to acute and chronic pulmonary hypertension. In this situation

- Diuretics may be given cautiously
- Relief of alveolar hypoxia with supplemental O_2 often improves ventricular function by reducing PAP
- Digitalis may be dangerous because of its potential for inducing serious arrhythmias in hypoxic patients

PRECIPITATING FACTORS

Factors that may have led to the acute worsening of the patient's respiratory condition are listed in Table 1. These factors should be considered in each patient, and specific treatment given in association with the above emergency therapy.

CRITERIA FOR INTENSIVE CARE ADMISSION

Patients with acute respiratory decompensation should be admitted to the intensive care unit if the following abnormalities are noted:

- Mental status
  - Progressive lethargy or actual coma
- Cardiac status
  - Arrhythmia or ventricular irritability
  - Hypotension
- Metabolic status
  - $Pa_{CO_2} > 65$ mm Hg and rising
  - Blood pH < 7.25 and falling
- Respiratory status
  - Labored breathing
  - Rapidly rising Pa_{CO_2}
  - Pa_{O_2} remains less than 40 mm Hg even on controlled supplemental O_2
  - Asynchrony of thoracic and abdominal respiratory muscles

TRACHEAL INTUBATION AND MECHANICAL VENTILATION

Indications for Tracheal Intubation in the CAO Patient

- Patient brought to emergency room in coma with CO_2 narcosis
- Rapid and/or steadily progressive rise in Pa_{CO_2}
- Rapid and/or steady fall in blood pH (usually below 7.25)

Mechanical Ventilation

When indicated, mechanical ventilation is initiated with tidal volumes of 7–10 cc/kg of body weight. The goals of therapy for the mechanically ventilated CAO patient include

- Ensure adequate oxygenation
- Improve V/Q by the measures described previously
- Gradually reduce the Pa_{CO_2} to a steady-state pH level by adjusting the minute ventilation
- Provide the exhausted patient sufficient rest, adequate nutrition, and sleep
- Permit fatigued respiratory muscles to rest by using the assist–control mode of ventilation

Weaning from the Ventilator

Weaning should begin when

- The patient's cardiovascular status is optimal
- *Active* infection has been treated
- The previously described goals have been achieved

Occasionally, the patient cannot be weaned from the ventilator because of the advanced state of lung damage (see Chapter 16 for a discussion of ventilatory assistance and complications).

BIBLIOGRAPHY

1. Albert RK, Martin TR, Lewis SW: Controlled clinical trial of Methylprednisolone in patients with chronic bronchitis and acute respiratory insufficiency. *Ann Intern Med* 92:753–758, 1980.
2. Aubier M, Murciano D, Viires N, Lecocuicy Y, Palacios S, Pariente R: Increased ventilation caused by improved diaphragmatic efficiency during aminophylline infusion. *Am Rev Respir Dis* 127:148–154, 1983.
3. Kawakami Y, Kishi J, Yamamoto H, Miyamoto K: Relation of oxygen delivery, mixed venous oxygenation, and pulmonary hemodynamics to prognosis in chronic obstructive pulmonary disease. *N Engl J Med* 308:1045–1049, 1983.
4. Nicotra MB, Rivera M, Awe RJ: Antibiotic therapy of acute exacerbation of chronic bronchitis. A controlled study using tetracycline. *Ann Intern Med* 97:18–21, 1982.
5. Snider GL (ed): *Clinics in Chest Medicine, Emphysema,* Vol 4. Philadelphia, WB Saunders, September, 1983.
6. Sturani C, Bassein L, Schiavina M, Gunella G: Oral nifedipine in chronic cor pulmonale secondary to severe chronic obstructive pulmonary disease (COPD)—Short- and long-term hemodynamic effects. *Chest* 84:135–142, 1983.
7. Blair GP, Light RW: Treatment of chronic obstructive pulmonary disease with corticosteroids. Comparison of daily vs. alternate day therapy. *Chest* 86:524–528, 1984.

CHAPTER 11

Asthma

Morgan D. Delaney

Asthma is a lung disorder characterized by intermittent, paroxysmal airflow obstruction due to bronchoconstriction and bronchial inflammation. A variety of stimuli may trigger an asthmatic episode; remission may occur spontaneously or only after bronchodilator therapy. Severe, acute asthma is life-threatening, even though it usually responds to initial bronchodilator therapy. It usually requires hospitalization and intensive therapeutic intervention. It can be fatal.

In assessing the patient with an acute asthmatic attack, the clinician must answer four questions:

- Does the patient definitely have asthma?
- How severe is the asthma attack?
- What "level" of treatment will be required?
- Is hospitalization necessary?

DIAGNOSIS

Many other diseases can mimic acute exacerbations of asthma. Some diseases that can present clinically with bronchospasm are listed in Table 1 along with features to assist in differentiating them from asthma.

History

Asthma is often first diagnosed in childhood or young adulthood; hence, the patient is often well acquainted with his diagnosis as well as

Morgan D. Delaney • Pulmonary Laboratory, Division of Pulmonary Diseases and Allergy, George Washington University School of Medicine and Health Sciences, Washington, D.C. 20037.

TABLE 1. Diseases That Mimic Asthma

Disease	Distinguishing clinical features
Acute pulmonary embolism	Pleuritic chest pain; hemoptysis; acute onset of dyspnea; may have abnormal chest film
Pulmonary edema	Enlarged heart; S3, S4 gallop rhythm; neck vein distension; peripheral edema; pulmonary rales; abnormal chest film
Upper-airway obstruction (e.g., epiglottis, goiter, tracheal tumor, or compression)	Stridor; may have pharyngitis with increased salivation
Carcinoid syndrome	Gastrointestinal symptoms; flushing; skin rash
Aspiration	History of impaired consciousness; infiltrates on chest film
Psychogenic dyspnea	No wheezing; hysterical personality

the signs and symptoms of an acute exacerbation. The most common symptoms are summarized in Table 2. These symptoms frequently develop after exposure to an identifiable stimulus. Common precipitating stimuli are listed in Table 3. The symptoms usually are episodic; an attack may spontaneously wax and wane in intensity. Episodic symptoms such as described above should always suggest asthma. Infrequently, the symptoms of an acute attack are subtle, consisting of no more than nocturnal or early-morning cough, unaccompanied by the complaint of dyspnea or wheezing.

Physical Examination

The physical examination usually reveals wheezing as the hallmark of turbulent airflow. However, some patients with severe obstruction may have very diminished breath sounds without wheezes and only prolonged expiration to indicate obstruction. Other physical findings present in severe obstruction are listed in Table 4.

TABLE 2. Symptoms in Acute Asthma

Chest tightness	Cough, usually nonproductive
Chest congestion	Noisy breathing
Breathlessness	Wheezing

TABLE 3. Common Stimuli Precipitating Acute Asthma Attacks

Viral upper-respiratory-tract infections	Air pollutants
Specific allergens	Sudden changes in weather
Drugs (acetylsalicylic acid, nonsteroidal anti-inflammatory agents)	Irritative dusts
	Emotional stress
Exercise	Aspiration of gastric secretions
Cold air	Noncompliance with prescribed medications
Strong odors and fumes	
Tobacco smoke	

Spirometry

The diagnosis of asthma is confirmed with pulmonary function testing. Spirometry reveals a reduced forced expiratory volume at 1 sec (FEV_1) as a fraction of vital capacity (FVC). This abnormality is at least partially reversed when the test is repeated after the patient inhales an aerosol dose of an adrenergic bronchodilator.

Chest X Ray

The chest x ray is not needed to diagnose asthma. However, when there is purulent sputum production or pleuritic chest pain, the chest x ray may help identify a concomitant process such as pneumonia.

TABLE 4. Clinical Features of Severe Asthma

Physical examination
  Abnormal vital signs
    (tachypnea, heart rate > 120, elevated blood pressure)
  Pulsus paradoxus > 20 mm Hg
  Use of accessory muscles of respiration
  Sternocleidomastoid muscle tenderness
  Intercostal and supraclavicular retractions
  Silent chest
  Alteration in state of consciousness
Spirometry
  Abnormal spirometry ($FEV_{1.0}$ < 800 ml)
Arterial blood gas
  Abnormal arterial blood gases
    (Pa_{O_2} < 60 mm Hg, Pa_{CO_2} > 40 mm Hg, pH < 7.35)

Sputum Examination

A wet prep or Wright's stain of sputum may confirm the diagnosis of asthma by showing Curschmann's spirals or Charcot–Leyden crystals or by demonstrating that the purulence is due to eosinophils, not neutrophils.

JUDGING THE SEVERITY OF THE ASTHMATIC ATTACK

After ascertaining the diagnosis of asthma, the physician must assess the severity of the attack. Acute exacerbations can range from mild bronchospasm that is promptly reversible to full-blown status asthmaticus during which the patient is initially unresponsive to usual therapy and may only respond to intensive and prolonged treatment.

The clinical parameters that frequently accompany a severe asthma attack are listed in Table 4. When the patient is in acute respiratory distress, these points should be particularly noted.

Spirometry

Spirometry provides an objective measurement of the severity of airflow obstruction. The degree of reduction in FVC, $FEV_{1.0}$, and FEF 25–75 correlates directly with the severity of the attack. The patient with very severe asthma may be so dyspneic, and moving so little air, that spirometry is impossible to perform.

When the spirometer is not available, a simple, hand-held device may be used to measure peak expiratory flow. Although highly dependent on maximal patient effort during early expiration, it has proven to be a dependable, if rough, guide to the severity of an acute asthma attack. It is not sufficiently objective to be used for measuring response to therapy.

Arterial Blood Gas

The arterial blood gas (ABG) measurement reveals the overall success of the lung in performing gas exchange. Airflow obstruction produces an imbalance of ventilation and perfusion, resulting in hypoxemia, which is directly proportional to the degree of obstruction. A Pa_{O_2} less than 70 usually signifies a severe attack. The hypoxemia, and other factors such as altered lung mechanics, trigger hyperventilation, which lowers the

Pa_{CO_2}, giving rise to respiratory alkalosis. Note that the Pa_{CO_2} falls with hyperventilation much more than the Pa_{O_2} rises, because CO_2 is more readily diffusible. A normal or elevated Pa_{CO_2} in a hypoxemic asthmatic in acute respiratory distress is a danger signal. It reflects deterioration in the level of alveolar ventilation below that necessary to eliminate CO_2 and indicates that the airflow obstruction is so severe that the muscles of respiration are unable to compensate. This rise in Pa_{CO_2} is accompanied by the development of an acute respiratory acidosis, and respiratory arrest may soon follow.

Arterial blood gases should be obtained in the asthmatic

- When clinical signs indicate a severe attack, in order to establish the need for supplemental oxygen (see Table 4)
- To confirm clinical deterioration in a severe attack
- To identify patients needing mechanical ventilatory assistance

Other Laboratory Factors

Laboratory data other than spirometry and ABG determination are not helpful in determining the severity of asthma. However, they may help identify the cause of the exacerbation and direct therapy. For example, an elevated white blood count and gram stain of sputum may help to identify an infection. An elevated hematocrit may suggest dehydration requiring more vigorous fluid replacement. Persistent blood eosinophilia may identify the atopic individual and suggest a role for corticosteroids.

TREATMENT

When the diagnosis of asthma is certain, the clinician must next determine the level of treatment required to achieve and maintain control of the attack. This depends on its severity. Only the therapy of an acute attack of moderate-to-severe asthma, and of status asthmaticus, will be considered here (see Fig. 1).

Oxygen and Nonpharmacologic Measures

Overall therapeutic measures to be employed during the severe acute attack of moderate-to-severe asthma are listed in Table 5.

Supportive measures include supplemental oxygen, hydration, avoidance of sedation, clearance of secretions, and endotracheal intubation for

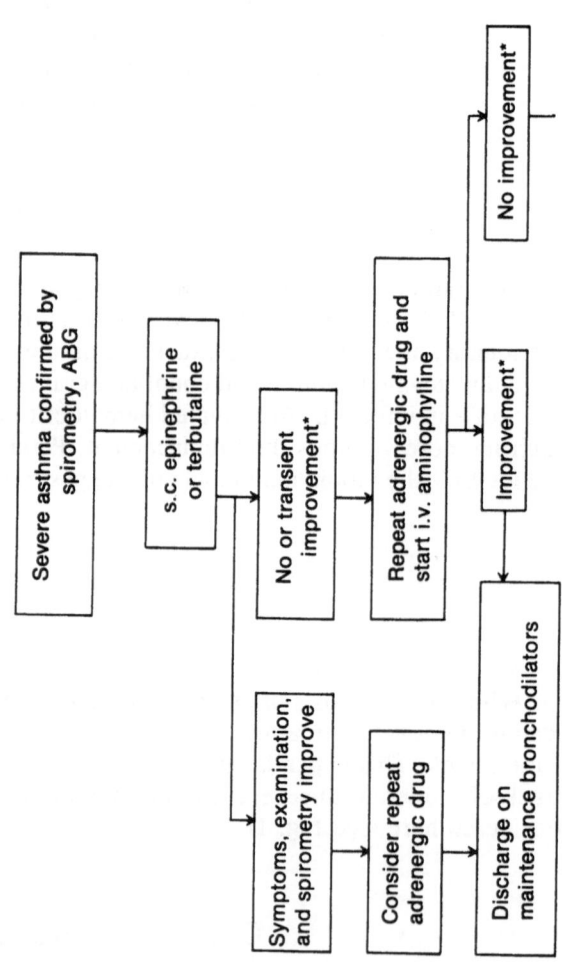

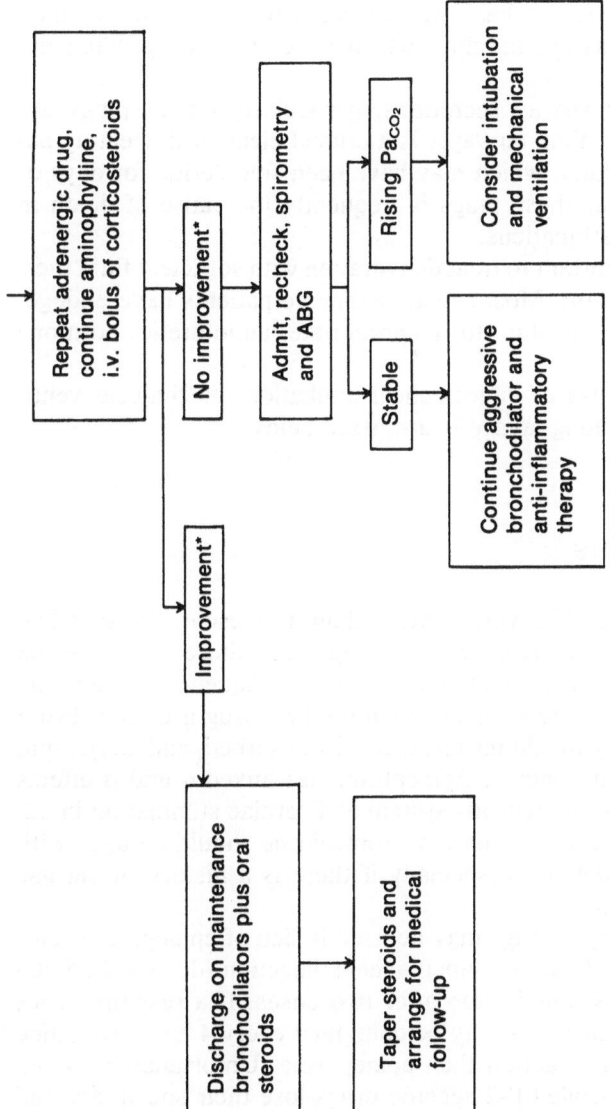

FIGURE 1. Algorithm for treatment of severe asthma. *, improvement refers to symptoms, examination, and spirometry or ABG.

mechanical ventilation. The specific measures include bronchodilator and corticosteroid therapy, which directly address the problems of broncho-constriction and bronchial inflammation and are discussed below.

Not all asthmatics require oxygen during an acute attack. The sensation of dyspnea may arise from pulmonary stretch receptors and occur with mild of no reduction in Pa_{O_2}. Hence, an ABG should be obtained before initiation of oxygen therapy, which is required only when the PaO_2 is below 70.

The clearance of airway secretions, particularly mucus plugs obstructing small and medium airways, is a critical element in treating patients with severe asthma, which may have been smoldering for days or weeks. Failure to clear these plugs is frequently the cause of death in patients with status asthmaticus.

Although it is important to treat dehydration with sufficient fluid therapy, avoid overhydration. Most severe asthmatic patients have endogenous volume expansion due to inappropriate antidiuretic hormone secretion.

The appropriate use of endotracheal intubation, mechanical ventilation, sedatives, and lung lavage is discussed below.

Sympathomimetic Agents

Parenteral Route. If severe acute asthma is present, the first line of therapeutic agents are the β-adrenergic agonists; these drugs are the most potent dilators of bronchial smooth muscle. Aqueous epinephrine 1:1000 (0.3–0.5 mg) has traditionally been the first drug used for severe acute asthma. It is easy to administer, is readily absorbed, and has a rapid onset of action, within minutes. Epinephrine has mixed α and β effects and thus results in central nervous system and cardiac stimulation in addition to its excellent bronchodilation. Epinephrine should be used with caution in elderly asthmatics especially if there is a history of cardiac disease or hypertension.

Other β-2 adrenergic drugs may be used in lieu of epinephrine. *Terbutaline sulfate* is available for subcutaneous injection (dose is 0.25–0.5 mg). If no response is noted, stop after two doses. If a response does occur, maintenance injections may be continued every 4 hr. Terbutaline has a longer duration of action than epinephrine. Unfortunately, when used parenterally, so-called β-2-specific drugs lose their specificity and usually cause significant central nervous system and cardiac side effects. Also, the bronchodilator effect of terbutaline is usually inferior to that of epinephrine.

Often the acute asthmatic attack can be reversed by simple injection of a parenteral adrenergic bronchodilator. The patient can then be sent home on his usual maintenance drugs; if he is not chronically taking med-

TABLE 5. General Outline of Therapeutic Measures for Severe Acute
Asthma

Supplemental oxygen
   Document hypoxemia with ABG
   Face mask or nasal cannula may be used to raise Pa_{O_2} to > 70 mm Hg
   Recheck ABG to assess adequacy of therapy
Adequate hydration
   Fluid may be given p.o. or i.v.
   Correct dehydration
   Maintenance administration of 3–5 liters of physiologic solutions each 24 hr
Mobilize lower-respiratory-tract secretions
   Maintain adequate hydration
   Encourage effective cough
   Chest physiotherapy if cough ineffective
Avoid sedation
Bronchodilator therapy
   Sympathomimetic agents
   Theophylline therapy
   Determine optimal dosage route
Corticosteroid therapy
Endotracheal intubation
   Mechanical ventilation
   Lung lavage
   Sedation, neuromuscular relaxation

ication, he should be instructed to begin using a metered-dose (MDI) inhaler of an adrenergic agent until the stimulus that provoked the acute attack has passed (see Table 8 for proper use of the MDI). It may be useful to administer an injection of Sus-Phrine (0.1–0.3 ml), an aqueous 1:200 suspension of crystalline epinephrine, which depends on its inso-lutility to provide a prolonged duration of action. Epinephrine in oil is another parenteral preparation with prolonged duration of action, but is not recommended because of unpredictable absorption.

Aerosol Route. Adrenergic bronchodilators may also be given by an aerosol route as initial treatment for acute asthma. Aerosol adminis-tration has been shown to have an onset of action within minutes, a pro-longed duration of effect of 4–6 hr, and usually more pronounced bron-chodilation than a comparable dose of the drug given orally or parenterally. In most cases, the aerosol route of administration is as ef-fective as the parenteral route.

However, in very severe attacks, the patient's markedly reduced minute ventilation impairs the delivery of an aerosol; in addition, the agitated patient may not be able to cooperate with aerosol administration. Hence, parenteral adrenergic therapy must be used.

Aerosols may be delivered effectively by a number of different de-vices, including MDI or a hand-held nebulizer. Intermittent positive-pres-sure breathing machines do not improve delivery of the aerosol. A variety

TABLE 6. Sympathomimetic Drugs for Parenteral Use in Acute Asthma in Adults

Drug	Initial dose	Immediate follow-up dose	Maintenance
Aqueous epinephrine (1:1000)	0.3–0.5 ml s.c.	0.3–0.5 ml s.c. q 30 min	—
Aqueous epinephrine suspension (Sus-Phrine) (1:200)	0.1–0.3 ml s.c.	—	0.1–0.3 ml s.c. q 6 hr
Epinephrine in oil (1:500)	0.2–0.5 ml i.m.[a]	—	—
Terbutaline sulfate (1 mg/ml)	0.25 mg s.c.	0.25–0.5 mg s.c. q 20–30 min ×2 only	0.25–0.6 mg q 4 hr

[a] Absorption can be unpredictable; this form of epinephrine is not recommended.

of β-agonist drugs are available as MDI, including racemic epinephrine, isoproterenol, metraproterenol, albuterol, and isoetharine. Currently available parenteral and inhaled solutions for use in treating asthma are listed in Tables 6 and 7. The proper use of an MDI (Table 8) must be demonstrated to the patient.

Asthmatics who have been using inhaled adrenergic drugs frequently prior to their visit to a physician for an acute attack may become relatively unresponsive to further administration of sympathomimetic agents. Sys-

TABLE 7. Sympathomimetic Drugs for Aerosol Use in Asthma in Adults

Drug	Volume of drug	Volume of saline diluent	Frequency of use
Solutions for use in hand-held or powered nebulizers			
Metaproterenol (5%)	0.2–0.3 ml	2–3 ml	q 4–6 hr
Isoetharine (1%)	0.25–0.5 ml	2–3 ml	q 4–6 hr
Isoproterenol (1:200/0.5%)	0.3–0.5 ml	2–3 ml	q 2–4 hr
Racemic epinephrine[a]	2–3 ml	None	2–3 inhalations q 15–30 min

Drug	Mg/puff	Puffs/use	Frequency
Metered-dose aerosols			
Bitolterol	0.37	2–3	q 6–8 hr
Albuterol	0.09	1–2	q 4–6 hr
Metaproterenol	0.65	2–3	q 3–6 hr
Terbutaline	0.2	1–2	q 4–6 hr
Isoetharine	0.34	1–2	q 3–4 hr
Isoproterenol[a]	0.125	1–2	q 3–6 hr
Epinephrine[a]	0.2	1–2	q 4–6 hr

[a] Routine use not recommended.

TABLE 8. Proper Use of Metered-Dose Inhaler

1. Shake the canister before use
2. Position the canister in front of the widely open mouth
3. Trigger the canister during the early part of a deep inhalation from residual volume to total lung capacity
4. Breath-hold at full inspiration for as long as is comfortable
5. Exhale through pursed lips
6. Repeat the procedure a second time with a 1- to 10-min pause between puffs
7. Inhaler should not be used more than 6–8 times within 24 hr

temic corticosteroids may need to be administered to restore the responsiveness of the β receptors.

Theophylline Therapy

Theophyllines are also useful in the treatment of acute asthma. Recent studies suggest that the adrenergic drugs discussed above promote more pronounced bronchodilation than aminophylline and thus are the first-line drugs. If the attack does not respond promptly to aerosolized or parenteral adrenergic drugs, then intravenous aminophylline is added. Adrenergic drugs have been shown to be synergistic with aminophylline. In addition to promoting bronchodilation, aminophylline is known to improve diaphragmatic contractility and delay diaphragmatic fatigue.

Before using aminophyline, it is important to establish whether the patient has been taking oral theophylline. If not, a loading dose of aminophylline is required. When the patient has been taken oral theophylline, the loading dose is reduced or eliminated and the maintenance infusion is instituted. Recommended loading doses and maintenance infusion rates are given in Table 9.

TABLE 9. Intravenous Aminophylline Therapy[a]

	Yes	No
Loading dose		
Has the patient been taking maintenance aminophylline as an outpatient?	0–3 mg/kg	6 mg/kg
Does the patient have evidence of a ventricular arrhythmia?	3 mg/kg	6 mg/kg
Maintenance dose		
Does the patient have heart or liver disease?	0.3 mg/kg per hour	0.6 mg/kg per hour
Does the patient have evidence of a ventricular arrhythmia?	0.3 mg/kg per hour	0.6 mg/kg per hour

[a] These are suggested doses and final dose should be adjusted on basis of theophylline blood levels.

If the aminophylline infusion is continued during subsequent hospitalization, it is essential to measure the plasma theophylline level to assess adequacy of therapy. The optimal theophylline blood level is 10–20 mg/ml; however, there is a great variation in individual tolerance of theophyllines. Many patients develop toxic manifestations at therapeutic or even subtherapeutic plasma levels. The most commonly observed adverse effects are nausea, vomiting, diarrhea, tachycardia, tachyarrhythmias, central nervous system excitation, and seizures. If adverse effects are suspected, the infusion should be discontinued and the plasma level measured.

Corticosteroid Therapy

Since the effects of corticosteroids will not be observed for several hours after administration, it is important to use them early in the treatment of the severe asthmatic. It is better to err on the side of overuse of steroids rather than to withhold them from the severe acute asthmatic in whom the response to initial therapy is uncertain; they can be rapidly tapered if found unnecessary later. Usually, the corticosteroids are given parenterally in a dose range of 100–250 mg of hydrocortisone equivalent every i.v. 4–6 hr. See Table 10 for specific indications for corticosteroid therapy in acute asthma.

If the patient ultimately improves enough to be sent home from the emergency room, and he has received corticosteroid therapy, the steroids should be continued orally in dosages of 20–60 mg of prednisone per day (as a single morning dose) until the patient is clearly stable, usually 4–7 days. Then the steroids are slowly tapered over 10–14 days.

Treatment to Avoid

Several medications, used in the treatment of chronic asthma, that have no role in the acute setting include

- Inhaled corticosteroids
- Inhaled cromolyn sodium
- Sedatives

TABLE 10. Indications for Corticosteroid Therapy in Acute Asthma

Status asthmaticus (absolutely mandatory)
An acute attack that is responding slowly to initial therapeutic interventions
History of chronic use of oral or inhaled corticosteroid preparations
Any asthmatic requiring hospitalization for the acute attack

In addition, avoid discharging severe, acute asthmatic patients from any emergency facility without making satisfactory arrangements for prompt *medical* follow-up. Many patients respond to acute measures only to relapse into subacute respiratory dysfunction at home.

WHO TO HOSPITALIZE

Three factors must be considered in deciding whether to admit the acute asthmatic to the hospital:

- The severity of the attack
- The speed of response to initial therapy
- The stability and severity of the patient's underlying asthmatic state

Signs of Impending Respiratory Failure

A severe attack, accompanied by any of the following signs of impending respiratory failure, demands admission:

- $Pa_{O_2} < 50$ mm Hg
- $Pa_{CO_2} > 50$ mm Hg
- pH < 7.35, whether respiratory or metabolic
- FVC < 1 liter
- Pneumothorax or pneumomediastinum
- Pulsus paradoxus > 20 mm Hg
- Altered state of consciousness

Ultimately, however, it is a clinical decision and no foolproof guidelines are available.

Objective Measurements of Improvement

Both laboratory and physical signs of respiratory distress subside as the attack improves. The physical signs that need to be monitored include

- Mental status
- Vital signs (blood pressure, pulse, respirations)
- Pulsus paradoxus
- Breath sounds
- Use of accessory muscles of respiration

In the patient with moderate or moderate-to-severe obstruction, abnormalities in the breath sounds are not a sufficient clinical parameter to follow because they reflect only the air movement in the medium and large airways where flow is turbulent. Breath sounds give no information about the small airways, which may be severely inflamed or plugged with mucus.

The most objective measurements of response to therapy are provided by repeating either spirometry or the ABG. It is important to measure objective parameters both initially and following therapy. Objective significant improvement must be present before discharge from the emergency room. If ABG were initially obtained, and were abnormal, they may need to be monitored serially.

Examples

When a chronically steroid-dependent asthmatic on maintenance bronchodilators presents with a severe acute exacerbation that responds slowly to treatment in the emergency room, he requires hospital admission.

The clinician should be particularly wary of the patient with multiple acute exacerbations, requiring emergency room or clinic care over the course of 7–10 days. This patient is likely to have marked mucus plugging and inflammatory changes of the small airways. The bronchospasm of the large airways may be partially reversed by parenteral therapy, making him feel better and sound better immediately. But this patient needs more prolonged intensive care to help clear the plugs and resolve the inflammation in the small airways. This patient is at risk for sudden death at home between emergency room visits.

When to Intubate

A few patients with status asthmaticus will develop severe respiratory failure and require mechanical ventilatory support. The indications for endotracheal intubation and mechanical ventilation are listed in Table 11.

TABLE 11. Indications for Tracheal Intubation and Assisted Mechanical Ventilation

Severe agitation requiring sedation to permit administration of therapy
Mental obtundation and coma
Progressively rising Pa_{CO_2} with a falling Pa_{O_2} and pH
Progressive clinical deterioration with obvious fatigue usually accompanied by a rising Pa_{CO_2} with a falling Pa_{O_2} and pH
Cardiopulmonary arrest

A few patients who are mechanically ventilated may also require lung lavage in an attempt to wash impacted mucus plugs out of the smaller airways so that effective alveolar ventilation can be achieved. After intubation and initiation of mechanical ventilation, it is often desirable to sedate the patient in order to relieve anxiety and agitation and reduce the disproportionate oxygen demands by the respiratory muscles. Sedation is only safe in treating acute asthma during controlled ventilatory assistance. Parenteral morphine sulfate is frequently used. Occasionally, neuromuscular blocking agents or even general anesthesia must be employed to achieve bronchorelaxation.

BIBLIOGRAPHY

1. Franklin W: Treatment of severe asthma. *N Engl J Med* 290:1469, 1974.
2. McFadden ER, Lyons HA: Arterial blood gas tensions in asthma. *N Engl J Med* 278:1027, 1968.
3. McFadden ER, Jr, Kiser R, De Groot WJ: Acute bronchial asthma: relation between clinical and physiologic manifestations. *N Engl J Med* 288:221, 1973.
4. Rebuck, AS, Read J: Assessment and management of severe asthma. *Am J Med* 51:788, 1971.
5. Rossing TH, Fanta CH, Goldstein DH, et al: Emergency therapy of asthma: Comparison of the acute effects of parenteral and inhaled sympathomimetics and infused aminophylline. *Am Rev Respir Dis* 122:365, 1980.
6. Vozen S, Kewitz G, Perruchoud A, et al: Theophylline serum concentration and therapeutic effect in severe acute bronchial obstruction: The optimal use of intravenously administered aminophylline. *Am Rev Respir Dis* 125:181, 1982.

PART IV

Pulmonary Vascular Emergencies

CHAPTER 12

Hemoptysis

Truvor Kuzmowych and Samuel V. Spagnolo

Severe hemoptysis, or pulmonary hemorrhage, is a life-threatening emergency. Indeed, hemoptysis regardless of its severity should always be considered a sign of serious pulmonary disease until proven otherwise. Literally, hemoptysis means to spit up blood, but in common usage it signifies coughing up blood.

DIFFERENTIAL DIAGNOSIS

Bleeding in the lung, from any cause, usually arises from a bronchial artery or an anastomosis between a bronchial artery and another systemic artery such as the intercostal. This explains the bright-red, arterial color of the blood. Rarely the bleeding source is entirely from the pulmonary circulation.

Table 1 provides a list of the common causes of hemoptysis. In spite of such a large differential diagnosis, a careful history (Table 2) and a thorough physical examination (Table 3), are extremely useful in narrowing the differential and reducing the number of laboratory tests necessary to confirm the diagnosis. For example, lung cancer would be very unusual as a cause of bleeding in a young child, because it is usually a disease of

Truvor Kuzmowych • Division of Pulmonary Diseases and Allergy, George Washington University School of Medicine, Washington, D.C. 20037; Pulmonary Clinic, Veterans Administration Medical Center, Washington, D.C. 20422. Samuel V. Spagnolo • Division of Pulmonary Diseases and Allergy, Department of Medicine, George Washington · University School of Medicine and Health Sciences, Washington, D.C. 20037; Pulmonary Disease Section, Veterans Administration Medical Center, Washington, D.C. 20422.

TABLE 1. Causes of Hemoptysis

Pulmonary infections	Neoplastic conditions
Bacterial	Bronchogenic carcinoma
Bronchitis	Bronchial adenoma
Bronchiectasis	Choriocarcinoma
Pulmonary tuberculosis	Metastatic osteogenic sarcoma
Lung abscess	Vascular conditions
Pseudomonas pneumonia	Pulmonary embolism with infarction
Staphylococcal pneumonia	Mitral stenosis
Klebsiella pneumoniae	Aortic aneurysm
Pulmonary actinomycosis	Arteriovenous fistula
Fungal	Primary pulmonary venous obstructive disease
Aspergillosis	Anomalous pulmonary vessels
Histoplasmosis	Miscellaneous
Coccidioidomycosis	Cystic fibrosis
Blastomycosis	Wegener's granulomatosis
Mucormycosis	Idiopathic hemosiderosis
Candidiasis	Goodpasture's syndrome
Parasitic	Pulmonary contusion
Paragonomiasis	Pulmonary laceration
Ancylostomiasis	Infected pulmonary cysts and bullae
Strongyloidiasis	Systemic lupus erythematosus
Echinococcosis	Vicarious menstruation
Schistosomiasis	Broncholithiasis
Ascariasis	Malingering

people over the age of 50. Information about the patient's place of residence, occupation, or travel may suggest parasitic or fungal disease as a likely cause of lung hemorrhage. Clubbing of fingers and toes points strongly to lung cancer in a man over 50, but in a young child, it raises the suspicion of primary cardiac disease. The volume of blood loss is also helpful in limiting the diagnostic possibilities (see Table 4).

In adults, the most common causes of pulmonary hemorrhage (in order of incidence) are tuberculosis (active or inactive), bronchiectasis, lung abscess, and carcinoma of the lung. In active tuberculosis severe bleeding is caused by rupture of a Rasmussen's aneurysm, which is an aneurysmal dilatation of a bronchial artery within a tuberculous cavity as a result of tissue necrosis. In inactive tuberculosis, bleeding is usually due to the colonization of a residual cavity in the lung by saprophytic organisms such as *Aspergillus* species, or other fungi, in the form of a mycetoma.

Less common causes of severe hemoptysis include

- Pulmonary contusion
- Bronchiectasis secondary to foreign body aspiration
- Rupture of aortic aneurysm into tracheobronchial tree
- Mitral stenosis
- Goodpasture's syndrome

TABLE 2. Historical Clues in the Diagnosis of Hemoptysis

Age (cystic fibrosis <30, carcinoma > 40)
Sex (vicarious menstruation in women)
Volume of hemoptysis (see Table 4)
Smoking history (carcinoma, bronchitis)
History of a heart murmur (mitral stenosis, aortic aneurysm)
Occupation (fungal infections)
History of anticoagulant ingestion
Geographic location or history of travel (fungal or parasitic infections)
Associated signs and symptoms, especially
   Weight loss (carcinoma, chronic infection)
   Night sweats (tuberculosis, lymphoma)
   Fever (infection)
   Chest pain (pulmonary embolism, infection with pleuritis)
   Bleeding from other sources (coagulopathy—Osler–Weber–Rendu)
History of kidney disease (Goodpasture's syndrome, Wegener's granulomatosis)
History of seizures or fainting (lung abscess)

TABLE 3. Clues from the Physical Examination in the Diagnosis of Hemoptysis

Naso- or oropharyngeal pathology (carcinoma, lung abscess)
Angiomata on skin and/or mucous membranes (Osler–Weber–Rendu)
Heart murmur (mitral stenosis, aortic aneurysm)
Clubbing of fingers (carcinoma, chronic infection)
Cyanosis (congenital cardiac disease)
Lymphadenopathy (carcinoma, chronic infection)
Blood in the stool (parasitic lung disease)
Copious and/or foul-smelling sputum (lung abscess, bronchiectasis)
Hoarseness (carcinoma)
Pleural friction rub (pulmonary embolism, infection, pleurisy)
Fever (infection)
Blood and/or protein in urine (Goodpasture's syndrome, Wegener's granulomatosis)

TABLE 4. Common Causes of Hemoptysis in Adults based on the Severity of Blood Loss per 24 hr

Mild hemoptysis[a]	Moderate hemoptysis[b]	Severe hemoptysis
<20 cc	>20 cc to <200 cc	>200 cc
Chronic bronchitis	Bronchiectasis	Tuberculosis
Lung cancer	Lung cancer	Bronchiectasis
Tuberculosis	Bronchitis	Lung abscess
	Tuberculosis	Lung cancer

[a] Usually only blood-streaked sputum.
[b] Frankly bloody sputum.

In children common causes of severe hemoptysis include bronchiectasis, cystic fibrosis, and bronchopulmonary sequestrations.

DIAGNOSTIC EVALUATION

Initial Evaluation

To conclude that the lung is the source of the coughed (or spit) up
blood, one must either visualize the bleeding site or exclude other possible
sites such as the upper airway, esophagus, and stomach.

Helpful clues to distinguish hemoptysis from hematemesis are listed
in Table 5. Hemoptysis, regardless of the amount of blood, should always
be investigated. In severe hemoptysis, the urgency of the situation must
not be allowed to compromise the completeness of the diagnostic evaluation. Tables 6 and 7 provide a guide for diagnostic evaluation of the
patient with hemoptysis.

To identify patients at greatest risk, quantitate the amount of bleeding
by collecting all blood coughed up by the patient prior to and after arrival
at the hospital.

Assessing the Urgency of Therapeutic Intervention

The severity of hemoptysis correlates best with the rate of bleeding,
i.e., the volume of blood loss per 24 hr. Blood-streaked sputum signifies
mild hemoptysis. Moderate hemoptysis consists of coughing up frankly

TABLE 5. Helpful Clinical Clues in Distinguishing Hemoptysis from
Hematemesis

Hemoptysis	Hematemesis
Coughed up blood is bright red and frothy	Vomited blood is dark red and never frothy
pH of coughed-up blood is alkaline	Vomited blood has an acid pH
Patient likely to have a history of chronic productive cough	Patient has a history of gastrointestinal disorders or chronic alcohol abuse
Microscopic examination shows RBC, WBC, microorganisms, pulmonary macrophages and possibly iron-filled macrophages	Microscopic examination may show food particles
Persistent flecks of blood in sputum produced after the acute episode	Sputum produced after the acute episode is clear of blood

TABLE 6. Initial Diagnostic Evaluation of the Patient with Hemoptysis

History
Physical
Chest x ray
Complete blood count, including
   Hemoglobin and hematocrit
   WBC and differential
   Examination of peripheral blood smear
   Platelet count
Complete urinalysis with microscopic examination of spun specimen
Prothrombin time, PTT, and/or bleeding time
Examination of sputum:
   Wet mount or Wright's stain
   Gram stain
   AFB stain
   Cytology
Arterial blood gas
Tuberculin skin test (PPD)

bloody sputum at the rate of less than 200 cc/24 hr. Severe hemoptysis, or pulmonary hemorrhage, is defined as coughing up blood at the rate of 200–600 cc (or more) per 24 hr.

Blood loss occurring at more than 200 cc/24 hr has the greatest potential for immediate life-threatening consequences. Although such a vol-

TABLE 7. Diagnostic Tests Used in the Workup of Hemoptysis and Some of Their Clinical Indications

Diagnostic procedure	Clinical indication
Laryngoscopy	Rule out laryngeal carcinoma
Bronchoscopy	Localize site of tracheobronchial bleeding
Technetium-labeled red blood cell scan	Localize site of tracheobronchial bleeding not seen on bronchoscopy
Bronchial, intercostal, and/or pulmonary angiography	Precisely localize site of bleeding and select arteries for embolization therapy; diagnose pulmonary embolism
Ventilation–perfusion scan	Diagnose pulmonary embolus or assess patient's ability to undergo resectional lung surgery
Tomograms and/or computerized tomography scan	Help visualize a mycetoma or carcinoma of the lung
Electrocardiogram and/or echocardiogram	Diagnose mitral stenosis, tricuspid endocarditis; help diagnose pulmonary embolus
Total eosinophil count	Help diagnose parasitic lung disease
Sputum and/or stool examination for ova and parasites	Diagnose specific parasitic lung disease
Fungal serologies	Help diagnose pulmonary fungal infection
Pulmonary function tests	Assess patient's ability to tolerate resectional lung surgery

ume is not large in proportion to the total intravascular blood volume, the cause of death in pulmonary hemorrhage most frequently is not exsanguination, but asphyxiation from blood clotting in the tracheobronchial tree. The volume of the entire tracheobronchial tree approximates the anatomic dead space of the lungs, about 150 cc. Therefore, an acute blood loss of only 200 cc into the lungs is an emergency because it can severely obstruct the airways and subsequently impair ventilation and gas exchange. Rarely, exsanguinating hemoptysis can occur when blood loss is at least 1000 cc, at a rate of 150 cc, or more, per hour, thus posing a threat to the patient's life from both asphyxiation and exsanguination.

Bronchoscopy

Who? Ideally, bronchoscopy should be performed in all patients with hemoptysis, and especially in patients with

- Hemoptysis for longer than 1 week
- An abnormal chest x ray
- A long history of cigarette smoking
- Age 40 years, or older

Why? Bronchoscopy is used to localize the site of bleeding and to establish a diagnosis. The shorter the period between the onset of hemoptysis and bronchoscopy, the greater the chance of identifying the bleeding site.

How? The type of bronchoscope used (i.e., rigid versus fiberoptic) depends on the skill and expertise of the bronchoscopist, as well as the amount and rate of hemoptysis.

In a severe pulmonary hemorrhage, the rigid bronchoscope is the preferred instrument because it not only provides an airway, but, at the same time, permits vigorous suctioning and allows the use of jet-ventilation to maintain respiratory gas exchange during the procedure.

Other Techniques Used to Localize the Bleeding Site

- Technetium-labeled red blood cell scan
- Bronchogram
- Pulmonary angiogram
- Selective bronchial and intercostal artery angiograms (this procedure should be done only when embolic therapy is planned)

THERAPY OF PULMONARY HEMORRHAGE

Goals

Treatment of the patient with hemoptysis consists of three primary goals:

- Maintain the airway
- Stop the bleeding
- Treat the underlying pathology

In mild-to-moderate hemoptysis, maintenance of the airway and stopping the bleeding are usually not a problem. The amount of blood loss is not large enough to cause major airway problems, and in most patients, the hemoptysis will spontaneously stop. The primary goal in such situations is to identify and treat the underlying pathology.

In severe hemoptysis, however, the volume and particularly the rate of blood loss are life-threatening, and for this reason the three primary goals of therapy frequently overlap. For example, it may be impossible to maintain an airway without slowing or stopping the hemorrhage first, and frequently, surgical resection will stop the bleeding while simultaneously removing the underlying cause. Management should depend on the patient and the resources available.

General Measures

While the diagnostic workup is in progress, initial therapy should consist of

- Patient reassurance
- Complete bed rest with the bleeding side down (when known)
- Judicious use of antitussives, for example, codeine, 30–60 mg every 4–6 hr

Care must be taken not to oversedate the patient since complete suppression of the patient's cough reflex may worsen gas exchange by promoting aspiration of blood. Any bleeding diathesis or coagulopathy must be corrected when possible.

When to Intubate

In severe hemoptysis when the above measures fail to decrease bleeding, intubation of the trachea may be necessary. Intubation may be done with a Carlens tube, which is a double-lumen endotracheal tube. This tube allows ventilation of the "good" lung with simultaneous isolation and suctioning of the bleeding lung. The Carlens tube is technically difficult to position in the trachea and should be inserted by an experienced person.

If the right lung is the source of bleeding, the left mainstem bronchus can be intubated with a single-lumen, cuffed endotracheal tube. When the cuff is inflated, this allows ventilation of the left lung and prevents spillover or aspiration of blood from the right lung.

When the site of bleeding is in the left lung, the left mainstem bronchus can be occluded with a large Fogarty catheter under bronchoscopic guidance. The trachea is then intubated with a single-lumen endotracheal tube to permit unimpeded ventilation of the right lung. The endotracheal tube must be placed well above the main carina and not into the right mainstem bronchus. The right mainstem bronchus is shorter than the left, and the inflated cuff of an endotracheal tube inserted into it can easily occlude the orifice of the right-upper-lobe bronchus.

Nonspecific Therapy

Endobronchial instillation of calcium oxalate or cobra venom is not effective in tracheobronchial hemostasis. The use of intravenous Pitressin or endobronchial iced saline lavage is controversial.

Medical Management

Medical management includes the therapeutic steps described previously, under General Measures. This conservative approach should be tried initially even when treating severe hemoptysis since it allows for

- Stabilization of the patient
- Time to obtain complete control of bleeding in the patient's airway with intubation and/or balloon tamponade
- Spontaneous cessation of the hemorrhage in up to 75% of patients

Nevertheless, with medical therapy alone, the mortality rate is between 25 and 50% in patients with severe hemoptysis. In addition, even if bleeding stops, recurrent bleeding occurs frequently. Situations where medical therapy alone is appropriate include patients with

- Bleeding due to pulmonary involvement of a systemic disease
- Bleeding due to diffuse and/or progressive pulmonary disease
- Minimal pulmonary function, who cannot tolerate a thoracotomy and lung resection

Surgical Management

Surgical therapy of pulmonary hemorrhage consists of a thoracotomy and excision of the segment, lobe, or entire lung from which the patient is hemorrhaging.

Who Should Be Operated On? Patients with pulmonary hemorrhage should be considered for surgical resection if they have sufficient pulmonary reserve to tolerate lung resection and have pulmonary disease that is localized to a specific segment or, at most, to one lung.

When to Operate? Mortality is over 30% for surgical therapy of severe hemoptysis without complete control of bleeding in the major airways. When bleeding in the major airways is controlled, the mortality of surgical therapy falls to 0–13%. Therefore, the best time to operate on a patient with pulmonary hemorrhage is after the major airway bleeding has been controlled or when the patient is not acutely hemorrhaging.

OTHER FORMS OF THERAPY TO CONTROL HEMOPTYSIS

Endobronchial Tamponade

Indications. Endobronchial tamponade therapy is used to control bleeding in patients who are not surgical candidates, but who continue to bleed with medical management. It is also helpful to control bleeding in patients prior to thoracotomy.

Technique. The segmental, or subsegmental, bleeding bronchus is first identified by fiberoptic bronchoscopy. The bronchus is then occluded with a Fogarty catheter and the bronchoscope is removed. The catheter is left in place for 1–2 days.

Arterial Embolization Therapy

Indications. Arterial embolization therapy can be used to control the bleeding in patients who continue to bleed with medical management and who may not be surgical candidates.

Technique. The thoracic aorta is first catheterized. Selective angiography is used to define the anatomy of the bronchial, spinal, and intercostal arteries at the bleeding site. In addition, a pulmonary angio-

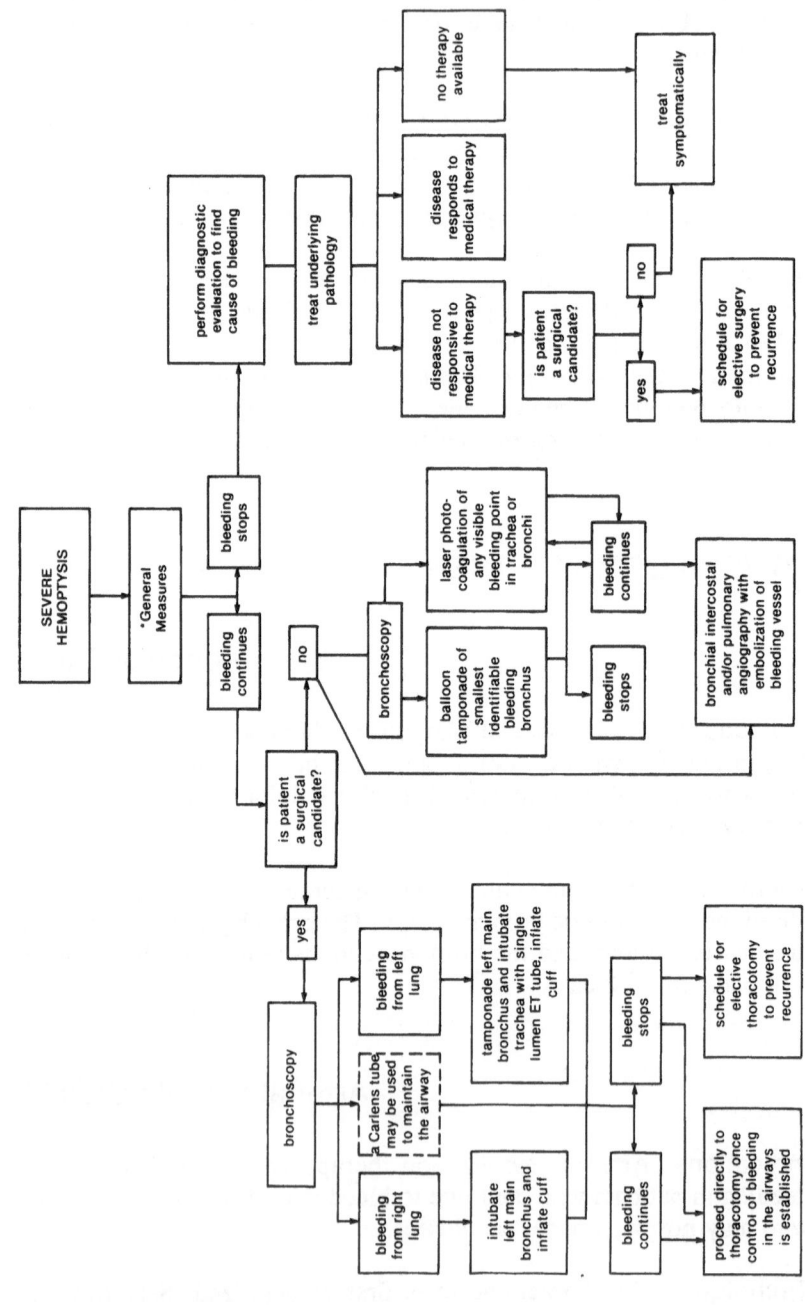

FIGURE 1. Algorithm for treatment of severe hemoptysis. *, See text for discussion.

gram may also be necessary. After the bleeding vessel is identified and selectively cannulated, it is occluded by injecting an absorbable gelatin sponge (Gelfoam) through the catheter.

Complications. Paraplegia can occur with arterial embolization therapy. Spinal arteries may arise from the bronchial or intercostal arteries that supply the bleeding vessels, and must be carefully avoided. Irritation, spasm, or occlusion of the spinal artery at this level, although uncommon, may result in infarction of the spinal cord with subsequent paraplegia.

Laser Photocoagulation

An effective and promising new technique for the control of bleeding from malignant tracheal or endobronchial lesions is laser photocoagulation administered through a fiberoptic or rigid bronchoscope.

SUMMARY

Patients with severe hemoptysis and localized lung pathology causing their bleeding should undergo thoracotomy with pulmonary resection to prevent future hemorrhage. Surgical therapy gives excellent results when complete control of bleeding in the patient's airways has been achieved, or when the patient is not acutely hemorrhaging at the time of thoracotomy. However, in patients who do not have localized lung disease, cannot tolerate a thoracotomy, or simply refuse surgery, endobronchial balloon tamponade, selective embolization of bronchial or intercostal arteries, and laser photocoagulation provide reasonable therapeutic alternatives when a trial of conservative management fails. This approach to treatment is summarized in Fig. 1.

BIBLIOGRAPHY

1. Arabian A, Spagnolo SV: Laser therapy in lung cancer. *Chest* 86:519–523, 1984.
2. Bobrowitz ID, Ramakrishna S, Shim YS: Comparison of medical v. surgical treatment of major hemoptysis. *Arch Intern Med* 143:1343–1346, 1983.
3. Crocco JA, Rooney JJ, Fankushen DS, DiBenedetto RJ, Lyons HA: Massive hemoptysis. *Arch Intern Med* 121:495–498, 1968.

4. Garzon AA, Cerruti MM, Golding ME: Exsanguinating hemoptysis. *J Thorac Cardiovasc Surg* 84:829–833, 1982.

5. Garzon AA, Gourdin A: Surgical management of massive hemoptysis. *Ann Surg* 187:267–271, 1978.

6. Gottlieb LS, Hillberg R: Endobronchial tamponade therapy for intractable hemoptysis. *Chest* 67:482–483, 1975.

7. Lyons HA: Differential diagnosis of hemoptysis and its treatment. *Basics RD* 5:2, 1976.

8. Stern RC, Wood RE, Boat TF, et al: Treatment and prognosis of massive hemoptysis in cystic fibrosis. *Am Rev Respir Dis* 117:825–828, 1978.

9. Uflacker R, Kaemmerer A, Neves C, et al: Management of massive hemoptysis by bronchial artery embolization. *Radiology* 146:627–634, 1983.

10. Yang CT, Berger HW, Conservative management of life threatening hemoptysis. *Mount Sinai J Med* 45:329–333, 1978.

CHAPTER 13

Embolic Pulmonary Disease

Aram A. Arabian

INTRODUCTION

Emboli from venous sources usually come to rest in the lungs and may cause subsequent damage to the heart, the lungs, or both. Commonly, the lungs and the heart are not involved in the primary thrombogenic process, but they become secondarily involved when emboli are trapped in the pulmonary vasculature. The types of emboli include thromboemboli, tumor emboli, foreign body emboli, air emboli, and fat emboli. The clinical presentation and the necessary treatment vary with the type of emboli. This chapter will concentrate on the most common—pulmonary thromboemboli (PE).

Incidence figures reveal more than 500,000 nonfatal and 50,000–150,000 fatal cases of PE per year. The embolus usually originates in a systemic vein, often the iliofemoral, and usually lands in the pulmonary circulation. Pathologic processes that lead to formation of thrombi are venous stasis, venous trauma, and changes in systemic coagulation leading to a hypercoagulable state. The size of the embolus and cardiopulmonary consequences determine the clinical presentation.

VENOUS THROMBOSIS

The most common cause of PE is deep venous thrombosis (DVT) of the lower extremity with subsequent embolization. The risk factors for

Aram A. Arabian • Division of Pulmonary Diseases and Allergy, George Washington University School of Medicine and Health Sciences, Washington, D.C. 20037; Respiratory Care, Veterans Administration Medical Center, Washington, D.C. 20422.

TABLE 1. Risk Factors for Venous Thrombosis and Pulmonary Embolism

Prior history of deep venous thrombosis
Heart disease
Cancer of the pancreas, lung, genitourinary tract, colon, stomach, breast
Trauma to the extremities, pelvis, spine
Surgery to the lower extremities, pelvis, spine
Pregnancy
Estrogen use
Immobilization
Obesity
Type A blood group
Deficiency of antithrombin III
Myeloproliferative disorders (polycythemia rubra vera, thrombocythemia, myeloid metaplasia)
Inflammatory bowel disease
Cushing's disease
Homocystinuria
Behçet's syndrome

DVT are the same as those for PE (see Table 1). Patients with a prior history of DVT are at the greatest risk for recurrence. Heart disease plays a significant role in the etiology of DVT, and all forms of heart disease, except hypertension, are associated with an increased risk of DVT. Cancer is an independent risk factor with carcinomas of the pancreas, lung, genitourinary tract, colon, stomach, and breast showing the greatest predeliction for DVT. Trauma to the lower extremities, pelvis, or spine is associated with an increased incidence of DVT, and the longer the immobilization, the greater the risk. Another form of trauma leading to DVT is that related to prolonged venous catheterization for parenteral hyperalimentation. The types of surgery with the greatest incidence of DVT are operations on the back, pelvis, and extremities. Pregnancy contributes to an increase in DVT, and delivery by cesarean section further increases the risk. Oral estrogen-containing compounds, whether used for contraception, suppression of lactation, or therapy for prostatic carcinoma, increase the risk of DVT, and the higher the estrogen dose, the greater the risk. Immobilization increases the incidence of DVT because of prolonged venous stasis. Obesity is associated with an increased incidence of DVT as measured by labeled fibrinogen scanning of the lower extremities. Those with a familial predisposition to DVT usually have a deficiency of antithrombin III.

Diagnosis of DVT

The complaint of leg pain, associated with calf swelling, warmth, and tenderness, suggests the presence of DVT. The standard method for confirming the diagnosis of DVT is venography, and the most reliable finding is an intraluminal filling defect. Noninvasive methods for diagnosis include impedence plethysmography (IP) and leg scanning with [^{125}I]fibrinogen. IP is usually done first, and if positive with clinical signs strongly suggesting DVT, treatment is instituted. False-positive IP testing may occur when there has been previous leg trauma or venous disease. When there is a strong clinical suspicion of DVT and IP is negative, it may be repeated after an interval of 1–3 days or fibrinogen leg scanning may be done; if either is positive, then treatment is indicated. Venography is used when clinical suspicion is low but IP and leg scanning are positive, or as a primary diagnostic modality when the latter are not available.

DVT Prophylaxis

Table 1 gives the risk factors for PE. Candidates for prophylaxis are patients with venous stasis or those who will be immobilized for an extended period. The most serious side effect of heparin prophylaxis is thrombocytopenia; hence, serial platelet counts must be monitored.

The incidence of DVT can be reduced by removing or reducing the risk factors. If this cannot be done, subcutaneous heparin, oral anticoagulants, or intravenous dextran should be used. Other, more controversial modes of prevention include treatment with intermittent leg compression, use of antiplatelet agents (other than dextran), and elevation of the foot of the bed 6–8 in.

The heparin dose used for prophylaxis is 5000 units administered subcutaneously every 8–12 hr. Dextran (10% of 40,000 or 6% of 70,000 average molecular weight) is administered in volumes of 500–1000 ml daily or every other day, given as a single infusion. For long-term prevention, oral anticoagulants are used and the dosage adjusted to maintain the prothrombin time at a level 1.5–2.5 times normal.

Although controversial, an inferior vena cava filter may be used prophylactically. It may be indicated in patients who are considered to be at prolonged, high risk for PE and who would probably not survive an acute embolic episode.

PULMONARY THROMBOEMBOLISM

Clinical Presentation

The most common presenting symptoms (reported in 60–90% of patients) are sudden onset of pleuritic chest pain, dyspnea, and apprehen-

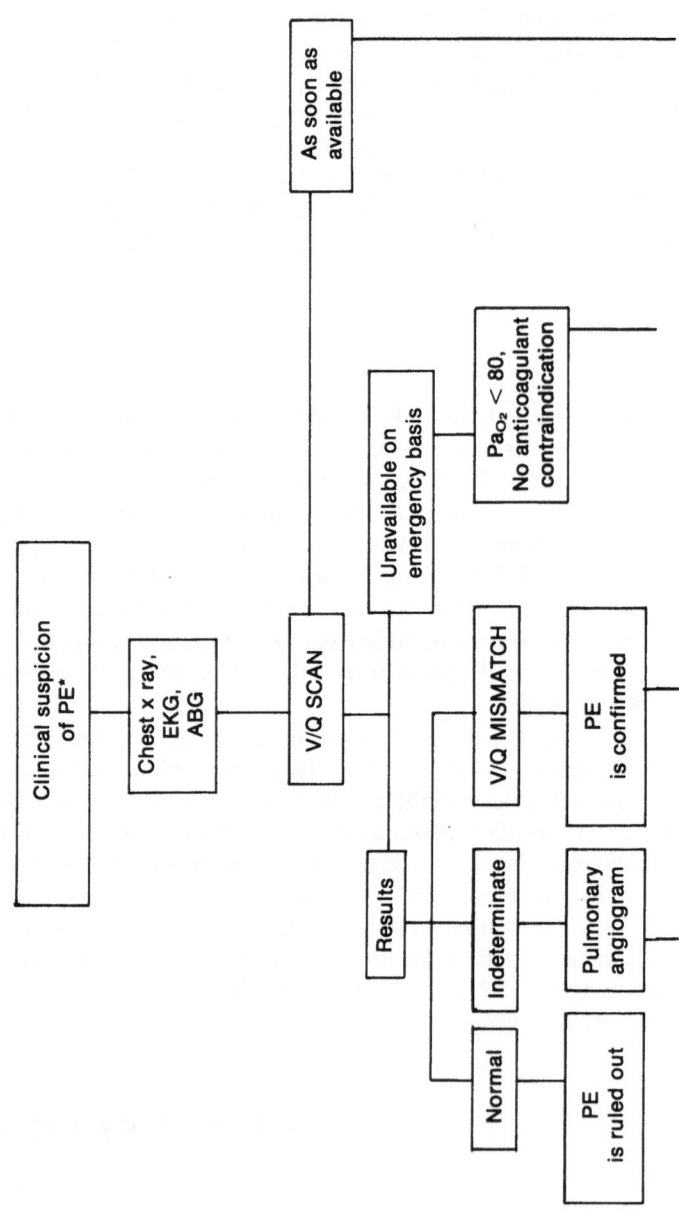

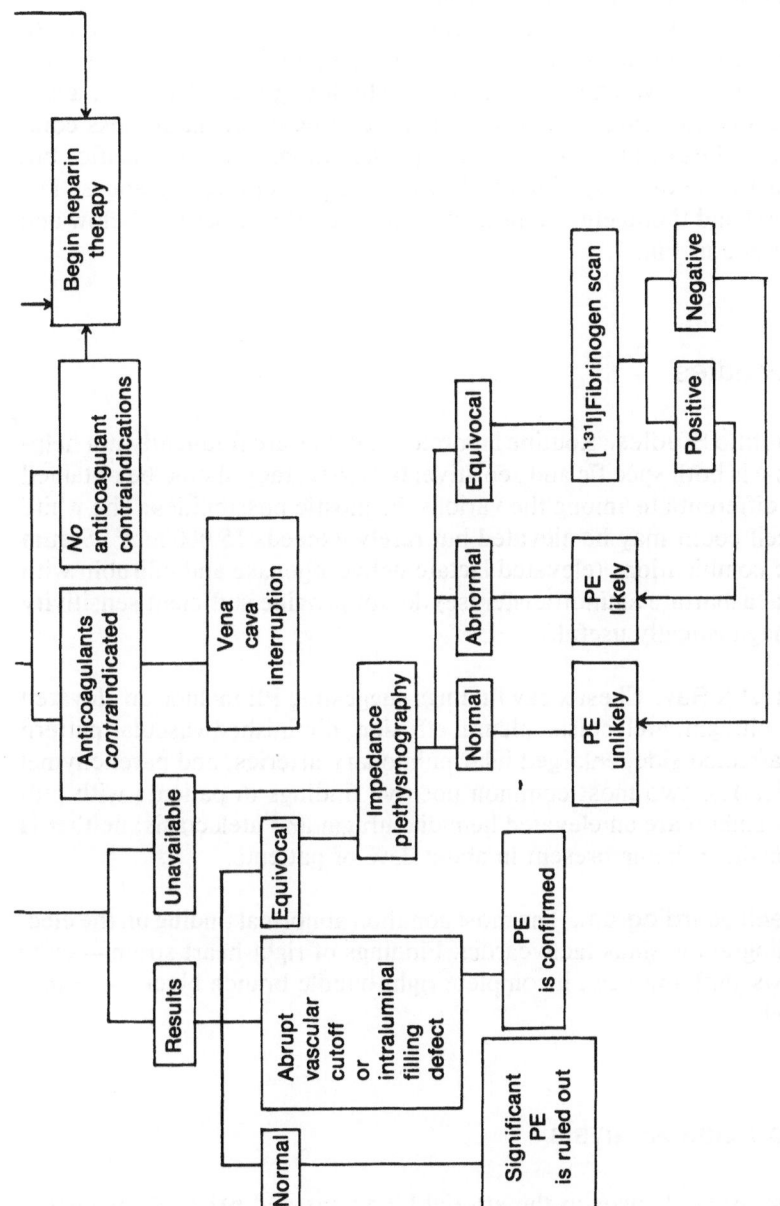

FIGURE 1. Algorithm for diagnosis of pulmonary embolism (PE). *, Refer to text for common presenting symptoms of pulmonary embolism (PE).

sion. Cough and hemoptysis are less common (reported in 30–50%). The symptoms of PE are nonspecific, but when risk factors for DVT are present, the diagnosis should be suspected. A significant number of patients have no detectable risk factors.

Common presenting signs (seen in 45–95%) are tachypnea (>16 breaths/min), rales, an increased pulmonic component to the second-heart sound, and an elevated temperature (usually low-grade). Phlebitis, a gallop rhythm, wheezing, diaphoresis, and peripheral edema are less commonly (25–35%) found. The clinical presentations are nonspecific, but they must raise the suspicion of PE given the proper circumstances. The diagnostic and therapeutic approach to the patient is described below and summarized in Fig. 1.

Laboratory Studies

Routine Studies. Routine laboratory studies are frequently not helpful. None is both specific and sensitive; however, they should be obtained to help differentiate among the various diagnostic possibilities. The white blood cell count may be elevated but rarely exceeds 15,000/mm^3. Serum enzyme combinations (elevated lactate dehydrogenase and bilirubin with a normal aspartate aminotransferase) do not provide sufficient sensitivity to be diagnostically useful.

Chest X Ray. Chest x-ray findings suggesting PE include an elevated hemidiaphragm, atelectasis, pleural effusion, diminished vascular pattern on the affected side, enlarged hilar pulmonary arteries, and parenchymal infiltrate. The two most common positive findings in patients with pulmonary emboli are an elevated hemidiaphragm and atelectasis; neither is very sensitive, being present in about 25% of patients.

Electrocardiogram. The most common abnormal finding on the electrocardiogram is sinus tachycardia. Findings of right-heart strain—acute right-axis shift and new, incomplete right bundle branch block—are rare (< 20%).

Arterial Blood Gas Analysis

The usual changes in the arterial blood gas and pH analysis (ABG) are alkalosis (pH > 7.44), hypoxemia (Pa_{O_2} < 80 mm Hg), hypocarbia (Pa_{CO_2} < 36 mm Hg), and an increased alveolar–arterial oxygen tension difference [$P((A\text{-}a)_{O_2}$ > 25]. The most sensitive ABG finding is the increased $P(A\text{-}a)_{O_2}$. It is rare for a patient to have a normal ABG during the acute episode. Although the specificity of this test is low, the sensitivity is quite high.

Other Tests. The more specific tests look for the presence of clot or evidence of arterial obstruction in the pulmonary vascular system. Tests to diagnose PE must be compared to pulmonary arteriography because, as yet, none is as specific.

Fibrinogen Degradation Products. Serum fibrinogen (or fibrin) degradation products (FDP) are often elevated in acute PE while normal in simple DVT. This is an indirect test that shows activation of the fibrinolytic system. However, FDP are normal in other diseases most often considered in the differential diagnosis—pneumonia, myocardial infarction, and bronchospasm. When elevated, correlation of FDP with diagnostic angiography has been good (better than 80%). FDP are also elevated in chronic liver and renal disease, in disseminated intravascular coagulation and systemic lupus erythematosus, and in patients receiving heparin therapy.

Ventilation–Perfusion (V/Q) Lung Scanning. The V/Q lung scan is most helpful in determining the absence of PE. Its greatest diagnostic value occurs when it is normal since this correlates well with negative pulmonary arteriography indicating no PE. Given the proper clinical circumstances, the V/Q lung scan is also diagnostic when ventilation-to-perfusion mismatches are found (V normal, Q abnormal in at least a multiple segmental distribution) indicating a probable PE. However, when less than segmental, perfusion abnormalities or matched defects are found, the interpretation must be correlated with the clinical presentation. Hence, there are three possible interpretations of a V/Q lung scan: normal, indeterminate, and mismatched. Normal and mismatched interpretations correlate highly with normal and positive arteriography. The indeterminate scans often require further testing. Unfortunately, patients with chronic airway obstruction, a pleural effusion, or a parenchymal infiltrate on chest x ray usually have an abnormal *baseline* V/Q scan, unrelated to PE. In these patients, the V/Q scan is likely to be indeterminate and less helpful in identifying PE; however, it may still help when there is a recent lung scan available for comparison, when there is mismatch in a lobar distribution, or when multiple segmental perfusion defects are present without ventilation defects.

When a pulmonary infarct develops, the V/Q scan will be indeterminate (matched V/Q defect) in the area of the infarct. If the scan shows mismatched perfusion defects in other areas, further diagnostic tests are not needed to confirm PE. However, if the only defects are matched, clinical judgement must determine how to proceed; the choices are to begin heparin or thrombolytic therapy or to perform pulmonary arteriography.

Pulmonary Arteriography. When less invasive studies have not determined the presence or absence of PE, pulmonary arteriography must be done. The diagnosis of PE is certain when there is an intra-arterial filling defect or an abrupt cutoff of a pulmonary artery. Finding a normal arteriogram does not guarantee against a prior PE, but probably means that the embolism was not clinically significant and does not require treatment. To be reliable, pulmonary arteriography requires high-resolution techniques and experienced angiographers.

Therapy

When there is a high index of suspicion of PE but the specific diagnosis cannot be readily obtained because emergency facilities for V/Q scan or arteriography are not available, therapy may begin with heparin and bed rest (unless thrombolytic therapy is needed—see below) until the diagnosis can be confirmed by further testing. However, a diagnosis based on clinical assessment alone is inadequate; objective data must be obtained before committing the patient to long-term anticoagulation.

Therapies available for PE (1) inhibit thrombi, (2) prevent emboli, (3) dissolve clots, or (4) mechanically remove clots. The indications and contraindications for each are different, and criteria for choosing one specific therapy over others are not universally accepted.

Heparin is an effective therapy for preventing clot propagation and allowing lysis and endothelialization of existing clot. Methods for administration of heparin include continuous and intermittent infusion. Table 2 gives a regimen for continuous infusion. The major complication of heparin therapy is hemorrhage.

Thrombolytic agents have recently become available, and their use has made surgical embolectomy unnecessary for acute, massive PE in most cases. Their use is indicated

- In massive pulmonary emboli (those obstructing the equivalent of two or more lobar pulmonary arteries)
- In submassive emboli with shock

Contraindications to the use of these agents are given in Table 3. Table 4 gives the doses for urokinase and streptokinase and Table 5 the laboratory monitoring required.

TABLE 2. Continuous Heparin Therapy

Loading dose: 5000–10,000 U
Continuous infusion: 1000 U/hr: modify infusion to maintain PTT[a] or LWCT[a] 1.5–2 times
  normal

[a] PTT, Partial thromboplastin time; LWCT, Lee White clotting time.

TABLE 3. Contraindications to Thrombolytic Therapy

Absolute contraindications
  Active internal bleeding
  Cerebrovascular process, disease, or procedure within 2 months
Relative contraindications (within 10 days of therapy)
  Major surgery, organ biopsy, or puncture of a noncompressible vessel
  Postpartum period
  Cardiopulmonary resuscitation with rib fractures
  Thoracentesis, paracentesis, or lumbar puncture
  Recent serious trauma
  Potentially serious bleeding
    Uncontrolled coagulation defects
    Uncontrolled severe hypertension
    Pregnancy near term

TABLE 4. Thrombolytic Dosages

Loading dose
  Streptokinase: 250,000 U over 20–30
    min
  Urokinase: 4400 IU/kg over 10 min
Maintenance dose
  Streptokinase: 100,000 U/hr for 24 hr
  Urokinase: 4400 IU/kg per hour for 12–
    24 hr

TABLE 5. Laboratory Monitoring of Streptokinase Therapy

Tests
  Whole blood euglobulin lysis time
  Thrombin time
  Partial thromboplastin or prothrombin time
  Fibrinogin degradation products
Before therapy
  Correct coagulation defects
  Determine baseline clotting study (if patient has been on heparin, use euglobulin lysis
    time or FDP to ensure thrombolysis)
After 3–4 hr of therapy
  Repeat baseline test to ensure fibrinolysis is occurring (thrombin time should be 2–3
    times normal)
If thrombolysis not confirmed
  Repeat loading and maintenance doses and recheck test
  If still no thrombolysis, begin urokinase or heparin

TABLE 6. Clinical Guidelines for Patient on
Thrombolytic Therapy

Minimize handling of the patient
Discontinue parenteral medications
Minimize invasive procedures
Apply compression bandages at sites of vessel punctures
Avoid concurrent anticoagulation and platelet-active drugs

When considering the use of thrombolytic agents, one must minimize trauma to the patient. Table 6 summarizes the guidelines to be followed during the use of thrombolytic therapy. This is a time when the patient has an increased risk of hemorrhaging, and for the 12–24 hr of therapy, all nonmonitoring, nonemergency procedures (including venipuncture) should be delayed. After the course of fibrinolytic therapy (when thrombin time is less than 2 times normal), heparin infusion must be given to prevent rethrombosis.

Inferior vena caval interruption or filtering is a treatment method that prevents emboli from the lower extremities from reaching the lung. Indications for this procedure include

- Patients with recurrent embolization from the lower extremities or lower vena cava that has proven refractory to anticoagulants
- Patients in whom anticoagulants are contraindicated
- Patients who develop serious complications from anticoagulant therapy

The Greenfield filter is an effective device for filtering the inferior vena cava. It can be inserted with a minor surgical procedure.

The indications for *surgical embolectomy* are not clear, since thrombolytic agents have become available. In the acute situation, thrombolytic agents are usually tried before surgery is considered. In the case of chronic pulmonary hypertension from recurrent PE, there may be a place for surgical removal of proximal clots in the pulmonary artery, since they usually do not respond to lytic therapy.

COMPLICATED PULMONARY EMBOLI

Pulmonary infarct and pneumonia may complicate PE. Pulmonary infarcts complicate about 10% of PE and occur when there is compromise of both the pulmonary and bronchial (systemic) circulations. They usually occur when there is obstruction of a small (<3 mm) branch of a pulmonary artery during a time when the systemic circulation is compromised, most often from congestive heart failure or shock.

Bacterial pneumonia may develop after PE. The clinical findings are similar to those of a bacterial pneumonia without PE and usually begin within a few days of the embolic episode. Therapy should include treatment for both PE and pneumonia. When hemoptysis occurs, the use of heparin or thrombolytics may impose a danger of increased hemorrhage, and a vena caval filter should be considered.

NONTHROMBOTIC PULMONARY EMBOLISM

Other types of emboli that can be trapped in the pulmonary vascular system are tumor emboli, septic emboli, air emboli, foreign body emboli, and fat emboli. Tumor emboli may metastasize to the lung but usually do not cause pulmonary or cardiac symptoms. Patients with septic emboli from a right-heart vegetation or a contaminated intravenous line often present with subacute, constitutional symptoms (fever, lethargy, anorexia); the chest radiograph showing multiple abscesses often leads to the diagnosis. Air emboli may be trapped in the pulmonary microcirculation causing stasis and leading to thrombus generation. If there are no paradoxic emboli, these usually resolve without sequelae. Foreign-body emboli usually present as an acute or subacute complication of an invasive intravascular procedure. Therapy requires extraction of the foreign body. Foreign-substance emboli from the intravenous injection of illicit drugs usually present as an acute-to-chronic disease, depending on the substance involved, and may cause a chest x-ray pattern ranging from pulmonary edema to bilateral lower-lobe interstitial disease. Fat emboli occur following long-bone fractures. They may cause simple obstruction of the pulmonary vasculature; however, a more serious condition often occurs 2–3 days later when the patient subsequently develops the adult respiratory distress syndrome (ARDS). Therapy is essentially that for ARDS (see Chapter 5).

BIBLIOGRAPHY

1. Bell WR: Pulmonary embolism: Progress and problems. *Am J Med* 72:181, 1982.
2. Fratantoni JC, Ness P, Simon TL: Thrombolytic therapy. *N Engl J Med* 293:1073, 1975.
3. Hyers TM (ed). *Clinics in Chest Medicine, Pulmonary Embolism and Hypertension*, Vol 5. Philadelphia, WB Saunders, 1984.
4. Moser KM: Pulmonary embolism. *Am Rev Respir Dis* 115:829, 1977.

5. Novelline RA, Baltarowich OH, Athanasoulis CA, et al: The clinical course of patients with suspected pulmonary embolism and a negative pulmonary arteriogram. *Radiology* 126:561, 1978.
6. Sharma GVRK, Cella G, Parisi AF et al: Thrombolytic therapy. *N Engl J Med* 306:1268, 1982.
7. Tsao MS, Schraufnagel D, Wang, NW: Pathogenesis of pulmonary infection. *Am J Med* 72:599, 1982.

CHAPTER 14

Superior Vena Cava Syndrome

Prashant Rohatgi

The superior vena cava syndrome (SVCS) is a clinical entity first described by William Hunter in 1757 in a patient with saccular aortic aneurysm. The SVCS is due to progressive obstruction of the superior vena cava by extrinsic compression or intrinsic thrombosis. This is a serious problem in clinical practice because it causes severe discomfort, is life-threatening to the patient, and requires prompt diagnosis and treatment by the physician.

ETIOLOGY

Bronchogenic carcinoma is the most common neoplasm producing this syndrome.

Major Causes of Superior Vena Cava Syndrome

Bronchogenic cancer	75%
Lymphoma	15%
Other metastatic malignancies	7%
Benign conditions	3%

It is estimated that 5% of all lung cancer and 15% of all cancers of the right upper lobe are associated with this complication.

Prashant Rohatgi • Pulmonary Disease Section, Veterans Administration Medical Center, Washington, D.C. 20422; Division of Pulmonary Diseases and Allergy, George Washington University School of Medicine and Health Sciences, Washington, D.C. 20037.

Many benign conditions can produce SVCS. These include intrathoracic goiter, idiopathic or granulomatous sclerosing mediastinitis, and superior vena cava thrombosis in association with intravenous central catheters.

CLINICAL SIGNS AND SYMPTOMS

The clinical manifestations of SVCS are related to the underlying disease and to the extent of obstruction of the venous drainage from the head and upper extremities. The constellation of signs and symptoms produced by superior vena cava obstruction is pathognomonic and can be easily recognized at the bedside.

Symptoms and signs of increased venous pressure include

- Dilation and tortuosity of the veins of the upper part of the thorax, neck, and arms
- Swelling and edema of the face, neck, upper extremities, and upper torso
- Flushing or cyanosis due to venous stasis
- Suffusion and edema of the conjunctiva, with or without proptosis
- Headache, dizziness, vertigo, distortion of vision produced by cerebral edema; in extreme cases, there may be convulsions, respiratory center disturbances, and depressed mentation including somnolence, stupor, and coma
- Hoarseness or stridor due to upper-airway obstruction caused by laryngeal edema and swelling of the tongue

DIAGNOSTIC APPROACH

The diagnosis of SVCS is made when the previously described signs and symptoms are noted. Confirmatory diagnostic procedures such as venography or digital angiography are rarely necessary to make the diagnosis (except when in situ thrombosis is suspected) and are usually not helpful in defining the histology of an obstructing tumor. It is important to establish a specific etiologic diagnosis of SVCS before treatment is initiated, except in patients with mediastinal widening on chest x ray and respiratory distress or far-advanced neurologic manifestations of cerebral edema because

- There is a significant, although low, incidence of benign diseases producing SVCS; in which case, empiric and unnecessary radiation may lead to long-term serious complications.

- The symptoms of SVCS are usually not rapidly progressive, as was formerly suspected, and most patients can tolerate a delay in therapy of 3–4 days to obtain tissue diagnosis without fatal consequences.
- Appropriate initial therapy may be important in determining the outcome of some of the major malignant causes of this syndrome, e.g., lymphoma and small-cell carcinoma.

CHEST X RAY

The usual radiographic abnormality seen in SVCS is widening of the anterior superior mediastinum, most commonly on the right side due to a space-occupying tumor in the path of the superior vena cava. Other abnormalities occur less often and include right hilar mass, right-upper-lobe collapse, anterior mediastinal mass, unilateral or bilateral hilar and paratracheal nodes, and pleural effusion. However, a *normal* chest x ray without mediastinal widening is still compatible with the diagnosis of SVCS if the other characteristic clinical findings are present.

COMPUTERIZED TOMOGRAPHY

Computerized tomography (CT) scan with intravenous administration of radiocontrast dye is sometimes useful in evaluating patients with SVCS. The CT scan may provide better delineation regarding the anatomic site, extent, and morphology of an obstructing lesion. The CT scan may show cystic changes, increased vascularity, or the presence of calcification in the obstructing lesion, which may narrow the differential diagnosis.

RADIOISOTOPE SCANNING

Patients suspected of having substernal thyroid or goiter on clinical examination or CT scan should have radioisotope scanning using ^{131}I or ^{99}Tc to confirm the location and extent of thyroid tissue.

VENOGRAPHY

Superior vena cava venography should be performed in patients with acute onset of SVCS who have central venous lines such as central venous catheters and pacemakers. In these patients, it is important to identify thrombosis around the central lines as the cause of obstruction of the SVC. Venography may also be necessary to confirm the diagnosis of SVCS in patients with a *normal* chest x ray.

BIOPSY PROCEDURES

Except for patients with thrombosis in association with central venous lines, most patients with acute onset of SVCS are likely to have an underlying malignant disease. These patients should be evaluated during the first 2 or 3 days with relatively safe procedures such as sputum cytology, biopsy of cervical, supraclavicular, or other palpable lymph nodes, and possibly bone marrow aspirate and biopsy. If these procedures do not yield a diagnosis, then fiberoptic bronchoscopy should be performed.

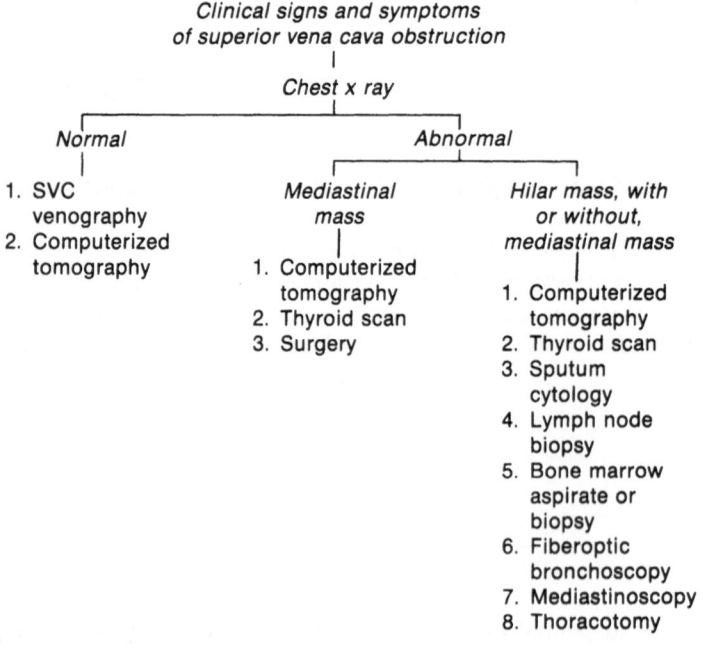

FIGURE 1. Schematic for diagnostic approach in superior vena cava (SVC) syndrome.

If bronchoscopy fails to reveal the diagnosis, then a choice should be made between mediastinoscopy and thoracotomy. Both procedures are likely to provide a definite diagnosis. However, the decision to perform mediastinoscopy should be tempered by the fact that the mediastinum in SVCS is filled with indurated and edematous tissue, which obliterates anatomic landmarks; in addition, bleeding may occur with the slightest surgical dissection and is difficult to control because of limited exposure of the surgical site. For these reasons, one should refrain from overzealous attempts to recover malignant tissue during mediastinoscopy. For a summary of the diagnostic approach in SVCS, see Fig. 1.

THERAPY

The basic therapeutic modalities in the management of SVCS are discussed in this section. The choice of therapy depends on the specific clinical situation and on the underlying etiology of the SVCS.

Empiric Radiation Therapy in Emergency Clinical Situations

For many years, empiric radiation therapy was recommended for SVCS of recent onset because catastrophic complete superior vena cava obstruction was considered imminent, most cases were due to malignant disease, and radiation was as effective as any available therapeutic modality in the treatment of inoperable malignant diseases.

Radiation remains the treatment of choice for SVCS associated with a wide mediastinum on x ray and evidence of rapidly progressive obstruction as suggested by the development of cerebral edema and upper-airway obstruction. In these situations, tissue diagnosis should be deferred so that immediate therapy can be given to alleviate the symptoms and to prevent respiratory failure and catastrophic cerebrovascular accident. Corticosteroids and diuretics are frequently used empirically as adjunct therapy under these circumstances to prevent or decrease edema.

Fibrinolytic and Anticoagulant Therapy

In case of rapid onset of SVCS in a patient with central venous catheter in place, the central lines should be removed and superior vena cava venography performed. If the diagnosis of superior vena cava thrombosis is confirmed, anticoagulants and fibrinolytic agents should be adminis-

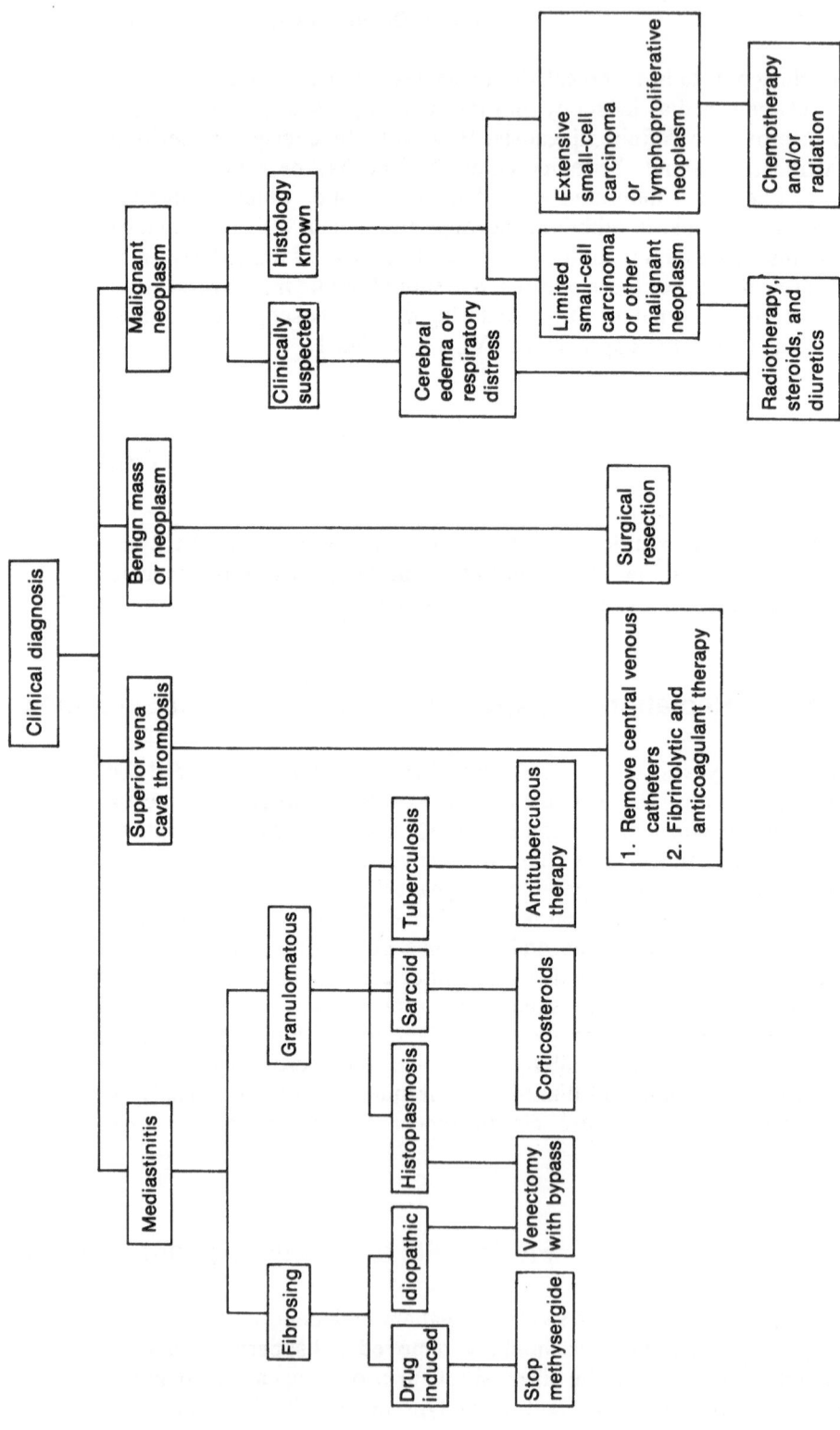

FIGURE 2. Therapeutic approach in superior vena cava syndrome.

tered following the standard guidelines and contraindications. (See Chapter 13.)

Radiation Therapy for Proven Malignancy

In general, initial radiation therapy consists of high-dose fractionation treatments of 300–400 rads in midplane for 3–4 days followed by a lower dose of 150–200 rads/day. The total dose is 3000–4000 rads for patients with malignant lymphoproliferative diseases and 5000–6000 rads for patients with epithelial malignant tumors. This is usually associated with symptomatic relief within 72 hr and is rarely associated with further compromise of the patient's condition from so-called "radiation edema."

Chemotherapy for Specific Malignancy

The results of current combined chemotherapy regimens have encouraged investigators to reconsider the value of radiation therapy as initial treatment for all tumor cell types. In stable patients with SVCS due to lymphoma or small-cell carcinoma, chemotherapy without radiotherapy may be preferred as initial treatment. This is particularly important in patients who have SVCS with tumor extending beyond a single radiation field.

Surgery

The role of surgery in the therapy of SVCS is limited and is confined primarily to patients with benign, space-occupying lesions compressing the superior vena cava. In an occasional patient, with fibrosing mediastinitis, bypass grafts of various types along with radical surgical excision have been employed to relieve venous obstruction. For a summary of the therapeutic approach in SVCS, see Fig. 2.

ADDITIONAL COMMENTS ABOUT MANAGEMENT

Venous Access Procedures

In view of the elevated venous pressures in the upper extremities in SVCS, venous access procedures in the upper extremities are likely to be associated with excessive bleeding. Similarly, because of the low flowrates in the upper extremities, intravenous or intramuscular drugs should be administered with caution in the upper extremities recognizing that the drugs will be slow to reach the systemic circulation and that the upper-extremity veins will be prone to thrombosis and phlebitis because of venous stasis. Whenever possible, venipuncture should be performed in lower extremities in these cases.

BIBLIOGRAPHY

1. Kane RC, Cohen MH, Broder LE, et al: Superior vena cava obstruction due to small-cell anaplastic lung carcinoma. Response to chemotherapy. *JAMA* 235:1717–1718, 1976.
2. Lakich JL, Goodman R: Superior vena cava syndrome. Clinical management. *JAMA* 231:58–61, 1975.
3. Mahajan V, Strimlan V, Vanordstrand HS, et al: Benign superior vena cava syndrome. *Chest* 68:32–35, 1975.
4. Painter TD, Karpf, M: Superior vena cava syndrome: Diagnostic procedures. *Am J Med Sci* 285:2–6, 1983.
5. Parish JM, Marschke RF Jr, Dines DE, et al: Etiologic considerations in superior vena cava syndrome. *Mayo Clinic Proc* 56:407–413, 1981.
6. Schraufnagel DE, Hill R, Leech JA, et al: Superior vena cava obstruction. Is it a medical emergency? *Am J Med* 70:1169–1174, 1981.

Pleural Emergencies

CHAPTER 15

Catastrophic Pleural Disease

Prashant Rohatgi

The accumulation of blood, serous fluid, pus, or air in the pleural space may result in a life-threatening situation for the patient. Prompt recognition and management are essential. This chapter will discuss each of these clinical situations separately.

CAUSES OF CATASTROPHIC PLEURAL DISEASE

Causes of catastrophic pleural disease include pneumothorax, tension pneumothorax, tension hydrothorax, hemothorax, and pleural empyema.

During normal (tidal) breathing, the lungs fill the chest so that the visceral pleura overlying the lung is in contact with the parietal pleura lining the thoracic cage. A potential "space" exists between these two layers of pleurae, and this "space" contains a small amount of fluid under subatmospheric pressure. The subatmospheric pressure is the result of expansile recoil of the chest wall and retractile elastic recoil of the lung. When air or fluid collects within this pleural space, the subatmospheric pressure becomes *less* negative or even becomes positive (higher than 1 atmospheric), and the lung retracts or collapses completely, whereas the chest wall expands.

The clinical manifestations of collection of air or fluid in the pleural space depend on

- The changes in gas exchange that occur with retraction or collapse of the lung

Prashant Rohatgi • Pulmonary Disease Section, Veterans Administration Medical Center, Washington, D.C. 20422; Division of Pulmonary Diseases and Allergy, George Washington University School of Medicine and Health Sciences, Washington, D.C. 20037.

- The hemodynamic consequences of increased or positive intrapleural pressure
- The nature of the fluid

Changes in Gas Exchange

With retraction and collapse of the lung the caliber of airways and pulmonary vessels decreases and the resistance of airways and pulmonary vessels increases. The collapse of the alveoli and increase in airway resistance leads to maldistribution of air and alveolar hypoxia. This results in active (reflex) pulmonary vasoconstriction with concomitant reduction in perfusion and thus minimizes ventilation–perfusion mismatching and the degree of arterial hypoxemia. (This is why the arterial hypoxemia in "simple" pneumothorax, defined below, is rarely severe except in patients with underlying lung disease and is often limited to the first several hours after a pneumothorax.)

Hemodynamic Consequences of Positive Intrapleural Pressure

Positive intrapleural pressure causes

- Complete collapse of ipsilateral lung
- Shift of mediastinum into the contralateral hemithorax
- Compression of contralateral lung
- Decrease in venous return to the heart, with a reduction in cardiac output, as a result of increased intrapleural and intramediastinal pressure
- Progressive hypoxemia and hypercapnia

These effects are most marked during expiration.

Nature of Fluid

This is discussed separately in the following sections.

PNEUMOTHORAX

Pneumothorax is defined as a collection of air within the pleural space. There are two etiologic categories:

- *Spontaneous pneumothorax* (primary or secondary)
- *Traumatic pneumothorax* (including iatrogenic)

Within each of these categories, the pneumothorax may be either uncomplicated (simple) or complicated.

Spontaneous Pneumothorax

Primary spontaneous pneumothorax occurs in apparently healthy individuals without underlying lung disease, whereas secondary spontaneous pneumothorax is considered to be present when there is evidence of intrinsic lung disease.

Mechanisms. Spontaneous pneumothorax may follow

- Rupture of a subpleural bleb or erosion of a subpleural pulmonary process through visceral pleura
- Dissection of air into the alveolar interstitium and extension along the bronchovascular interstitial space into the lung hilum and mediastinum (pneumomediastinum); from this point it may dissect further into the neck, producing subcutaneous emphysema, and/or rupture through the visceral pleura producing pneumothorax

Traumatic Pneumothorax of Iatrogenic Variety

This can follow surgical procedures in the

- Neck, e.g., translaryngeal aspirate, throat surgery
- Thorax, e.g., needle aspiration of lung or pleural space, transbronchial lung biopsy, subclavian vein catheterization
- Abdomen, e.g., liver biopsy

They all produce pneumothorax by penetrating visceral pleura or by having air dissect along the fascial planes. Positive-pressure ventilation may produce barotrauma and cause pneumothorax by rupture of a subpleural bleb or dissection of air into the alveolar interstitium, as described before.

Noniatrogenic Posttraumatic Pneumothorax

This may follow penetrating or blunt chest injury. Penetrating injuries may produce either a closed pneumothorax by puncturing visceral pleura or an open (communicating) pneumothorax by permitting air into the pleural cavity directly through the chest wall. Most pneumothoraces are

a result of blunt chest trauma and are of the closed type. Blunt trauma
may produce closed pneumothorax by

- Laceration or puncture of the lung by the tip of a fractured rib or
  clavicle
- Dissection of air into the alveolar interstititum as a result of increased intra-alveolar pressure caused by compression of the chest
  wall with the glottis closed
- Rupture of the esophagus or by tear of the tracheobronchial tree
  by deceleration injury

Clinical Signs and Symptoms of Pneumothorax

The clinical presentation of pneumothorax will depend on its extent
and on the presence of underlying disease. The sudden onset of chest
pain, usually pleuritic in type, along with dyspnea is the most common
presenting symptom pattern. Persistent cough, hemoptysis, and syncope
are prominent manifestations in a few patients. Common physical findings
include tachypnea and shallow respirations. On the side of the pneumothorax, thoracic examination reveals chest hyperexpansion, splinting,
diminished respiratory excursion, diminished-to-absent vocal fremitus
and breath sounds, and a tympanitic percussion note. Five percent of
patients with pneumothorax are asymptomatic and have a normal chest
examination. Mediastinal emphysema is often detectable on auscultation
by the presence of a "crunching" or "popping" sound with each heart-
beat. The presence of cervical subcutaneous emphysema can be easily
recognized by its characteristic crepitation on palpation of the neck.

Diagnosis

Since the most common symptoms are dyspnea and chest pain, pneumothorax may be confused with pleurisy, pulmonary embolism, pneumonia, myocardial infarction, and rarely an acute abdominal condition.

The definitive diagnosis of pneumothorax is made by chest x ray. See
Fig. 1 to determine the size of the pneumothorax. A small pneumothorax
may be obscured when the chest roentgenogram is taken at full inspiration. In suspicious cases, an expiratory chest x ray should be obtained
to enhance the contrast between compressed lung and pleural space air.

Classically, the chest x ray in a pneumothorax shows the separation
of the visceral pleura from the parietal pleura by air in the pleural cavity.
The visceral pleura usually appears as a thin, convex line beyond which
one cannot see any bronchovascular markings. In addition, other abnormalities may be noted, such as blebs on the surface of the collapsed lung,

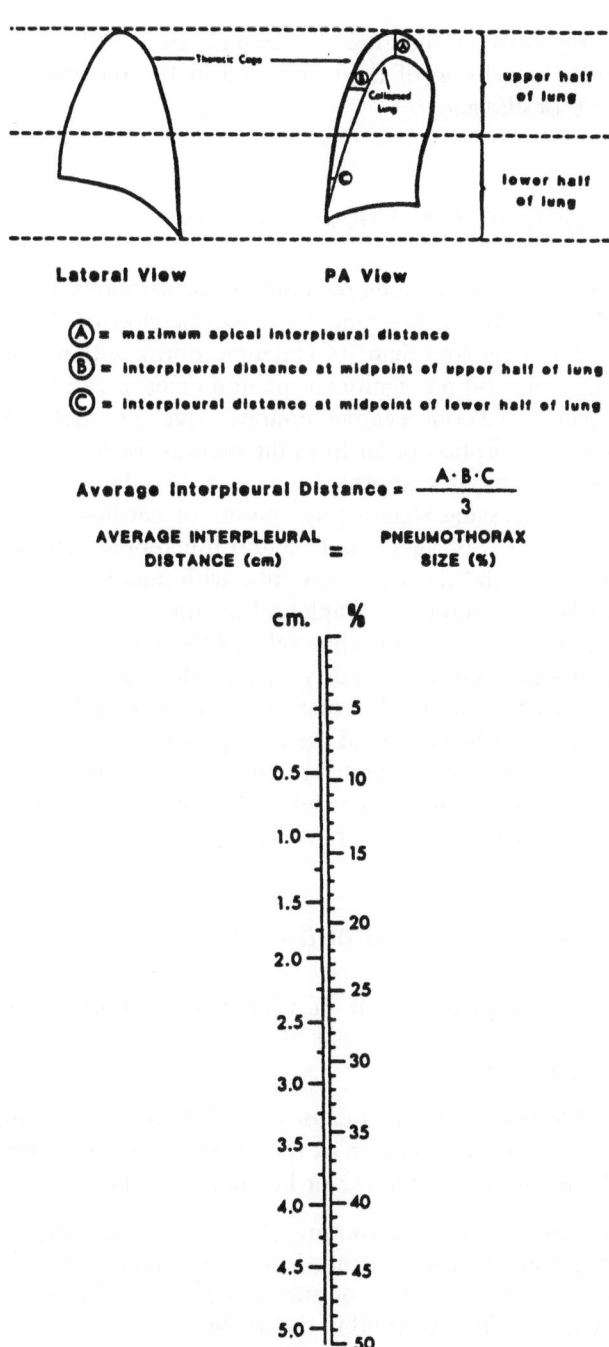

FIGURE 1. Determining the size of pneumothorax. Calculation of intrapleural distance and prediction of pneumothorax size. From Rhea et al., *Radiology* 144:733–736, 1982. Reprinted with permission.

pleural adhesions between the lung surface and chest wall, a hydropneumothorax due to collection of fluid or blood in the pleural space, and fracture of a rib or clavicle.

Management of Spontaneous Pneumothorax

In patients with spontaneous pneumothorax without complications, the principles of treatment are aimed at re-expansion of the collapsed lung. Patients who have less than 20% pneumothorax with no distressing signs and symptoms and no significant pleural disease can be managed, if followed closely, by a conservative, nonoperative approach, which permits spontaneous resorption of air from the pleural space. Some patients cannot be managed by this approach because of a large or increasing pneumothorax, distressing signs or symptoms of cardiovascular or gas exchange compromise, or significant pleural thickening. These patients need a closed intercostal thoracostomy tube with underwater seal drainage. Both needle aspiration of intrapleural air on a one-time-only basis and the placement of a narrow intrapleural catheter (16-gauge intravenous type) have been suggested as alternative therapeutic maneuvers. Although needle aspiration and catheter placement are attractive in their simplicity, accidental puncture or laceration of the re-expanding lung by needle and clogging of the needle and catheter are frequent complications. Thoracostomy tube drainage is *mandatory* when a spontaneous pneumothorax is complicated by hemopneumothorax or pyopneumothorax.

Management of Traumatic Pneumothorax

The emergency management of traumatic pneumothorax (closed type) is fundamentally similar to that of spontaneous pneumothorax except that one has to look for

- A possible tear in the trachea or proximal right or left main bronchus, or esophageal rupture as the cause of the pneumothorax
- Development of hemothorax or hemopneumothorax

A tear in the major airways or rupture of the esophagus should be suspected in the presence of uncontrolled pneumothorax, tension pneumothorax, mediastinal emphysema, or subcutaneous emphysema. Hemoptysis or unusual bleeding from within the trachea suggests a tracheal tear, whereas the presence of food particles in the pleural space suggests esophageal rupture. Patients suspected to have a tracheal or bronchial tear require bronchoscopic examination. Patients suspected to have esophageal rupture should initially have an x-ray examination of the esophagus following Gastrografin swallow, and if that study is negative, it should be followed by study with barium swallow. If either of the above injuries is found, or if the patient has evidence of significant bleeding within the pleural cavity, an immediate thoracotomy is necessary.

TENSION PNEUMOTHORAX

Tension pneumothorax is due to the development of the "ball valve" pleural leak; the visceral pleural leak seals when intrapleural pressure is positive during expiration and reopens when the pressure is relatively negative during inspiration. This causes continued collection of more air in the pleural space with each breath. This condition leads to progressively positive intrapleural pressure that not only totally collapses the affected lung, but also shifts the mediastinum into the contralateral lung with impedance to venous return. This produces the gas exchange and hemodynamic consequences discussed previously and leads rapidly to severe hypoxemia, hypercarbia, and cardiovascular collapse.

Clinical Signs and Symptoms of Tension Pneumothorax

Except for clinical evidence of mediastinal shift (tracheal deviation and the shift in the cardiac impulse to the contralateral side) and decreased cardiac output (tachycardia and reduced blood pressure), the clinical signs and symptoms of tension pneumothorax are exaggerated but the same as those described for uncomplicated spontaneous pneumothorax. As tension pneumothorax progresses, the patient develops increasing apprehension, agitation, labored breathing, increasing air hunger, cyanosis, elevated jugular venous pressure, weak, thready pulse, hypotension, and shock, which may be preceded by pulsus paradoxus.

Management

Tension pneumothorax can be rapidly progressive and fatal and requires emergency decompression of the pleural space. Occasionally, it is not possible to await definitive confirmation of the diagnosis with a chest x ray or to wait for ideal management by tube thoracostomy. In this emergency situation, a large-bore (16- to 18-gauge) needle attached to a three-way stopcock and a 50-ml syringe can be used for aspiration of air. The needle is inserted into the second anterior intercostal space, approximately three fingersbreadth lateral to the sternal angle on the side of the tension pneumothorax. Following emergency needle aspiration of a tension pneumothorax, the patient should be evaluated with chest x ray and treated with a closed intercostal thoracostomy tube with underwater seal drainage.

TENSION HYDROTHORAX

Tension hydrothorax is due to massive pleural effusion, which produces lung collapse and mediastinal shift, and like tension pneumothorax, it causes life-threatening impairment in gas exchange and hemodynamic compromise. Tension hydrothorax is extremely rare, and the pathogenesis of continued fluid accumulation despite an increase in hydrostatic pressure within the pleural cavity is incompletely understood. Most cases of tension hydrothorax are due to malignant pleural effusion.

Clinical Signs and Symptoms of Tension Hydrothorax

The onset of tension hydrothorax is not sudden, and there is invariably a prior history of pleural effusion. Clinical signs and symptoms are similar to those of tension pneumothorax except for the physical findings on chest examination on the side of the hydrothorax. The affected hemithorax shows hyperexpansion and diminished respiratory excursion with absence of both breath sounds and vocal fremitus. However, the most characteristic finding is dullness to percussion throughout the affected hemithorax. These patients also have pulsus paradoxus and elevated jugular venous pressure.

Differential Diagnosis

Since most cases of tension hydrothorax occur in patients with underlying malignancy, superior vena cava syndrome and cardiac tamponade must be distinguished from tension hydrothorax as more common causes of impaired venous return and impaired cardiac output.

Definitive Diagnosis

The definitive diagnosis of tension hydrothorax is made by

- Chest x ray, which shows opacification of the affected hemithorax with shift of the mediastinum to the contralateral side

- Thoracentesis, which demonstrates the presence of a pleural effusion on the affected side.

Management

The emergency treatment of tension hydrothorax is prompt decompression by performing thoracentesis and removing as much fluid as is necessary to relieve the symptoms. It is very important not to completely drain the pleural cavity since this may result in the development of *life-threatening* re-expansion pulmonary edema in the previously collapsed lung.

Pleural fluid obtained during initial thoracentesis should be sent for laboratory evaluation to establish the underlying etiology.

If tension hydrothorax recurs, the patient may require drainage with a thoracostomy tube and obliteration of the pleural space by intrapleural instillation of tetracycline or another sclerosing agent.

HEMOTHORAX

Hemothorax is defined as collection of blood in the pleural cavity. It may be life-threatening primarily because of blood loss from the intravascular compartment. Rarely does it lead to life-threatening hemodynamic consequences with impairment of gas exchange, as seen with tension pneumothorax or tension hydrothorax. In a small proportion of patients, hemothorax, especially when moderate, infected, or associated with injury to the pleura, may progress to form a fibrous peel around part or all of the lung. This peel may result in reduced lung function.

Etiology

Hemothorax is most commonly caused by trauma producing contusion of visceral or parietal pleurae, avulsion and laceration of pleurae at the site of adhesion, or puncture and laceration of the lung due to a protruding rib fracture or due to laceration of an intercostal or internal mammary artery. Iatrogenic hemothorax may follow attempts at percutaneous puncture of the subclavian vein. Hemothorax may follow anticoagulation in patients with pulmonary embolism and infarction. Occasionally, rupture of a dissecting aneurysm of the thoracic aorta produces a hemothorax, which is usually on the left side.

Clinical Signs and Symptoms

The signs and symptoms of hemothorax are those of pleural effusion, and when the bleeding is moderate to massive, the patient may exhibit signs of acute intravascular volume depletion such as hypotension or postural hypotension with tachycardia.

Differential Diagnosis

Pleural effusion developing after trauma may also be due to chylothorax from thoracic duct rupture and hydrothorax from esophageal rupture or pleural effusion associated with pancreatitis.

Definitive Diagnosis

Diagnosis of hemothorax requires

- X-ray evidence of pleural effusion with or without a fractured rib
- Finding blood on thoracentesis

When blood is aspirated, it is important to be sure that it represents a "true" bloody effusion and not a traumatic thoracentesis. A simple bedside test is to observe the fluid for clot formation. Blood obtained because of traumatic thoracentesis will clot within several minutes, whereas a "true" bloody pleural effusion that has been present for several hours will not clot in the test tube, because it has already clotted on formation in the pleural space, undergone fibrinolysis, and become defibrinogenated. Another simple test to differentiate true bloody effusion involves centrifuging the aspirated fluid. Fluid from a traumatic thoracentesis will yield a clear supernatant, whereas presence of icteric or xanthochromic supernatant indicates that blood was present in the pleural cavity for several hours.

Another problem in the evaluation of hemothorax is differentiation of a primary hemothorax from a primary serosanguineous effusion. In hemothorax, the hemoglobin concentration of the fluid is usually greater than 25% of that in the blood, whereas it is unusual for a serosanguineous effusion to have a hemoglobin concentration that exceeds 1.0 gm/dl.

Management

There is considerable controversy regarding proper management of hemothorax. It is prudent to remember two important principles:

- Bleeding from low-pressure blood vessels of the pulmonary circulation is likely to stop spontaneously, whereas bleeding from high-pressure blood vessels such as systemic arteries is likely to continue.
- Small amounts of blood are readily absorbed from the pleural space without any residual adverse effects.

Patients with uncomplicated minimal hemothorax, as evidenced by obliteration of the costophrenic angle, do not require active intervention because fluid will generally be resorbed within 10–14 days. A moderate hemothorax, which fills about one-third of the hemithorax, requires immediate and complete drainage along with replacement of intravascular volume. Repetitive thoracentesis with a large-bore needle should only be tried if one can completely evacuate the pleural cavity; otherwise, continuous closed-chest tube drainage should be utilized.

A large hemothorax, which fills half or more of the hemithorax, is indicative of bleeding from a systemic artery. In these cases, replacement of blood and closed-chest tube drainage is mandatory, preferably with two tube thoracostomies, one placed anteriorly and high and the other placed posteriorly and low. Thoracotomy for control of the bleeding vessel is required in these patients if brisk bleeding persists and blood transfusions are required to maintain an adequate hematocrit and blood pressure.

PLEURAL EMPYEMA

Pleural empyema literally means collection of "pus" in the pleural space; however, it is probably more practical to define it as "an infected pleural exudate."

The evolution of a pleural space infection from an adjacent bacterial pneumonia (parapneumonic effusion) can be divided into three pathologic stages, which merge imperceptibly into each other. The initial stage, the *exudative stage*, is characterized by rapid outpouring of thin, serous, exudative and sterile pleural fluid, with relatively low white cell count. At this stage, the patient responds to antimicrobial therapy, either alone or combined with needle aspirations. The second stage, the *fibrinopurulent phase*, is characterized by invasion of pleural fluid by bacteria and transformation of fluid to fibrin-rich purulent exudate, with loculation. At this stage, it is usually not feasible to drain the pleural space with needle aspiration alone, and generally, thoracostomy tube drainage with breaking of the loculations or rib resection with large thoracostomy tubes is required for effective drainage of pus. The final stage is the *organization stage*, in which fibroblasts grow into the exudate both from the visceral and parietal pleurae and envelop the lung in an elastic membrane, "the peel." At this stage, thoracotomy with decortication may be required to free the entrapped lung. If untreated, the empyema may drain spontaneously through the chest wall (empyema necessitans) or into the lung and produce a bronchopleural fistula.

Empyema is most commonly caused by adjacent bacterial pneumonia. However, it may also follow

- Penetrating thoracic injuries, either traumatic or iatrogenic, to the thorax
- Transdiaphragmatic spread of infection from a subphrenic abscess
- Contiguous spread from a paravertebral abscess, osteomyelitis of rib, or purulent mediastinitis
- Ruptured esophagus (generally this empyema is on the left side)
- Hematogenous seeding of the pleural space from a distant suppurative site

Clinical Signs and Symptoms

The clinical signs and symptoms of empyema are not diagnostic except to direct attention to the chest and to suggest an infectious process. Almost all patients have fever (>100.4°F). Some patients are critically ill with high fever and obvious signs of sepsis. Clinical signs and symptoms that specifically suggest pleural space disease include pleuritic chest pain, pleural friction rub, and physical findings of a pleural effusion.

Definitive Diagnosis

It is apparent from the discussion of the natural history of pleural space infections that the prognosis and therapeutic approach to parapneumonic effusion is largely determined by the stage in which the disease is recognized. Ideally, therefore, in patients with parapneumonic effusions one must balance the need to avoid unnecessary tube thoracostomies in patients who can be managed conservatively with antibiotics and needle aspiration as in the exudative stage, with the need to start tube drainage of the pleural space as early as possible in patients suspected to be in the fibrinopurulent stage of disease, because drainage becomes progressively more difficult the longer it is delayed. Thus, the aim in the diagnosis and management of parapneumonic effusions is the ability to predict which of the exudative effusions are likely to resolve with conservative treatment and which of the effusions are likely to progress to complicated stages of fibrinopurulent or fibrotic reaction.

Clinical and chest x-ray features are generally not useful in separating *uncomplicated* parapneumonic effusion from *complicated* parapneumonic

TABLE 1. Clinical Features and Pleural Fluid Characteristics Indicative of Complicated Bacterial Parapneumonic Effusions

---

Clinical features
    Presence of loculated fluir or air–fluid levels within the pleural space
    Rapid reaccumulation of fluid after thoracentesis
    Failure of parapneumonic effusion to respond to antibiotics
Pleural fluid characteristics
    Grossly purulent fluid
    Putrid odor
    Demonstration of bacteria on Gram stain
    Glucose < 60 mg/dl
    pH is less than 7.00 except in *Proteus* infection

---

effusion. However, the presence of the clinical features and pleural fluid characteristics listed in Table 1 suggests progression to complicated stages of parapneumonic effusion and requires complete evacuation of the pleural cavity.

The pleural findings that suggest that no further diagnostic or therapeutic measures are needed for management of parapneumonic pleural effusion are (1) pleural fluid pH above 7.20 (note the *Proteus* exception); (2) pleural fluid glucose above 60 mg/dl; and (3) pleural fluid lactate dehydrogenase below 1000 IU/liter.

The pleural fluid findings are considered to be indeterminate when (1) pleural fluid pH is between 7.00 and 7.20; (2) LDH level is above 1000 IU/liter in the absence of a large number of red blood cells; and (3) pleural fluid glucose is between 40 and 60 mg/dl. In these borderline cases, the need for thoracostomy tube drainage is determined by (1) the size and rapidity of accumulation of fluid and (2) the direction of change in serial pleural fluid samples obtained at 12- to 24-hr intervals.

Management

The management of complicated parapneumonic pleural effusions or pleural empyema consists of two parts: (1) appropriate antibiotic therapy depending on the organisms identified on Gram stain and culture of the pleural fluid or the organisms recovered from the contiguous or distant foci of infection thought to be responsible for empyema and (2) complete drainage of the pleural cavity by closed or open drainage.

Closed Drainage

Since the fluid in empyema may be viscous and loculated, closed drainage with thoracostomy tube should be attempted. A thoracostomy tube of as large a diameter as possible should be placed in the most dependent area of fluid accumulation. During tube insertion, an attempt should be made to break the loculations with a finger. In loculated effusions, more than one thoracostomy tube drainage may be necessary. The tube should be left in place until the purulent drainage disappears and the amount of serous drainage decreases to less than 75 ml/day, when it should be gradually withdrawn and removed.

Open Drainage

When closed thoracostomy tube drainage is not effective in clearing the pleural cavity, then either a rib resection with thoracotomy drainage or formation of an Eloesser flap—pleural cutaneous fistula—may be required.

Decortication

Occasionally after the empyema is controlled with closed or open drainage, there may be a residual organized peel enveloping the lung. In these circumstances, it may be necessary to decorticate and remove the organized peel so that the lung can expand and function normally.

BIBLIOGRAPHY

1. Light RW: Management of parapneumonic effusions. *Arch Intern Med* 141:1339–1341, 1981.
2. Getz SB Jr, Beasley WB III: Spontaneous pneumothorax. *Am J Surg* 145:823–827, 1983.
3. Rhea JT, DeLuca SA, Green RE: Determining the size of pneumothorax in the upright patient. *Radiology* 144:733–736, 1982.
4. Teplick SK, Clark RE: Various faces of tension pneumothorax. *Postgrad Med* 56:87–92, 1974.
5. Kirsh MM, Sloan H: Traumatic pneumothorax and hemothorax. in Kirsh MM, Sloan H (eds): *Blunt Chest Trauma. General Principles of Management.* Boston, Little, Brown, pp 49–79, 1977.
6. Samson PC: The intrapleural sequelae of chest injury, in Daughtry DC (ed): *Thoracic Trauma.* Boston, Little, Brown, pp 69–78, 1980.
7. DeSouza R, Lipsett N, Spagnolo SV: Mediastinal compression due to tension hydrothorax. *Chest* 72:782–783, 1977.

PART VI

Ventilator Emergencies

CHAPTER 16

Ventilatory Assistance and Its Complications

Aram A. Arabian, Ann Medinger, and Samuel V. Spagnolo

INTRODUCTION

Ventilatory emergencies occur when individuals are unable to ventilate their pulmonary gas-exchanging units adequately to meet metabolic needs. Preceding chapters have reviewed specific clinical respiratory emergencies that may require artificial mechanical ventilatory support when patients are critically ill. Whether the source of gas exchange impairment lies in airway obstruction, parenchymal infiltrate, vascular occlusion, pleural disease, or neuromuscular weakness, the final common pathway is ventilatory failure, which can be readily detected in the arterial blood gas (ABG). The Pa_{CO_2} rises above 44, pH falls below 7.36, and the Pa_{O_2} falls below age-predicted or previously stable values.

Assisted mechanical ventilation is lifesaving in the treatment of ventilatory failure. Although it is an integral part of advanced life support following cardiopulmonary resuscitation, it is most helpful to initiate mechanical ventilation *prior to* ventilatory collapse. To do this one must recognize the signs of impending collapse, which may develop over hours

Aram A. Arabian • Division of Pulmonary Diseases and Allergy, George Washington University School of Medicine and Health Sciences, Washington, D.C. 20037; Respiratory Care, Veterans Administration Medical Center, Washington, D.C. 20422. Ann Medinger • Division of Pulmonary Diseases and Allergy, George Washington University School of Medicine and Health Sciences, Washington, D.C. 20037; Pulmonary Function Laboratory, Veterans Administration Medical Center, Washington, D.C. 20422. Samuel V. Spagnolo • Division of Pulmonary Diseases and Allergy, Department of Medicine, George Washington University School of Medicine and Health Sciences, Washington, D.C. 20037; Pulmonary Disease Section, Veterans Administration Medical Center, Washington, D.C. 20422.

or days to weeks. The history, physical examination, and ABG yield the most useful information about ventilatory failure; the signs and symptoms, which vary with the different disease processes, have been reviewed in the preceding chapters. Progressive deterioration in the ABG clearly warns of ventilatory failure. Serum electrolytes may also provide a clue; an increasing anion gap (AG) may fortell increasing lactate from progressive respiratory muscle failure:

$$AG = Na^+ - (Cl^- + HCO_3^-)$$

This chapter will review the principles of mechanical ventilation, advantages of various ventilators, considerations in gaining access to the airway for ventilation, methods of initiating, adjusting, and discontinuing mechanical ventilation, and the potential complications of mechanical ventilation.

AIRWAY ACCESS

Mechanical ventilation requires access to the patient's tracheal airway. This is accomplished with either an endotracheal tube (inserted through nose or mouth) or a tracheostomy tube (inserted surgically through the neck). When upper-airway obstruction is the cause of the ventilatory failure, simple intubation of the airway may solve the problem without the need for mechanical ventilation. Except in pediatric patients, positive-pressure mechanical ventilation requires a tracheal tube with an inflated balloon cuff to prevent retrograde airflow around the airway and out of the patient. It is desirable to allow a small leak of air around the balloon cuff to minimize the pressure of the balloon on the tracheal mucosa.

Tracheal tube complications are minimized by checking the following items:

- Prior to intubation
  - Choose the largest tube compatible with the patient's anatomy.
  - Choose a tube with low-pressure cuff; check balloon for leaks.
- After intubation
  - Check the chest x ray for placement of the tube tip at least 1.5 cm above the carina and balloon below the vocal cords.
  - When inflating the balloon, allow a small leak of air around the balloon. (Detected by auscultation over the trachea and measurement of an expired volume 50–100 ml less than inspired.)

PRINCIPLES OF MECHANICAL VENTILATION

The purpose of the mechanical ventilator is to provide an adequate minute ventilation to gas-exchanging units ($\dot{V}_A$) without requiring any muscular effort from the patient. In most current ventilators, this is accomplished by blowing a volume of air (approximating a normal tidal volume) into the lung and then allowing passive deflation on a cyclic basis (aproximating a normal respiratory frequency). With such a device, one can potentially control the frequency of the cycles (F), the oxygen enrichment of the air (F_{IO_2}), the volume of air delivered (V_T), the flow rate, and the airway pressure. While all the ventilators discussed below allow control of the F_{IO_2} and F, control of the other factors varies from one type of ventilator to another and will be further discussed below.

The overall minute ventilation ($\dot{V}_E$) is simply calculated from the frequency of respiratory cycles (F) and the volume delivered with each cycle (V_T):

$$\dot{V}_E = V_T \times F$$

The $\dot{V}_E$ is an important factor to consider whenever adjustments are made in the mechanical ventilator, because it correlates best with the ABG. Measurement of the ABG will determine whether $\dot{V}_E$ must be increased, decreased, or maintained. The ventilator measurements of airway pressure and volume will determine whether V_T or F should be changed to achieve the desired $\dot{V}_E$.

The minute ventilation that actually reaches gas-exchanging units ($\dot{V}_A$) can be calculated by subtracting the volume of each breath that does not reach areas of gas exchange, called dead space (V_D):

$$\dot{V}_A = (V_T - V_D) \times F$$

In normal lungs, V_D is about equivalent in milliliters to ideal body weight in pounds. In the diseased lung, V_D often increases and may need to be measured. Increasing the tidal volume delivered by a ventilator increases the $\dot{V}_A$ more efficiently than increasing F. Hence, when the patient requires more $\dot{V}_A$, the V_T should be increased first if possible.

Lung and chest wall compliance are also important factors in mechanical ventilation. Compliance (C) is the elasticity of the lung and/or thorax, and it expresses the relationship between the volume of lung inflation and the pressure required to achieve that volume:

$$C = \Delta V/\Delta P$$

Lungs that are stiff because they are full of interstitial or alveolar fluid or fibrosis have a low compliance and require much higher pressures to inflate to a given volume. Hence when $\dot{V}_A$ must be increased to improve gas exchange, V_T should be increased first, *as lung compliance permits*. However, some patients with very stiff lungs cannot tolerate large V_T because of the high pressure required and risk of barotrauma. (See Complications of Mechanical Ventilation.) They must have F increased to raise $\dot{V}_A$.

CHOOSING A MECHANICAL VENTILATOR

The most common types of mechanical ventilators are pressure-cycled, volume-cycled, and time-cycled. These machines are named by the factor that determines the point of transition from the inspiratory to expiratory phase of each respiratory cycle.

Pressure-Cycled Ventilator

The pressure-cycled ventilator delivers a volume of air under positive pressure. Each cycle of inflation (or inspiration) ends when a preset pressure is reached, at which point passive expiration follows. Pressure is the control setting and the volume delivered is dependent on the compliance of the lung and chest wall. It is this maximal pressure that determines the volume delivered. If the lung is compliant, V_T may be high, but if compliance begins to fall, V_T and hence $\dot{V}_E$ may fall without warning. In some pressure-cycled ventilators, exhaled volume is measured and an alarm may warn of decreasing exhaled volumes. The pressure-cycled ventilator is not recommended for treating patients with cardiopulmonary instability because $\dot{V}_E$ cannot be accurately and consistently regulated.

Volume-Cycled Ventilator

The volume-cycled ventilator also delivers a volume of air under positive pressure followed by passive expiration. However, in this machine volume is the control setting, and the pressure generated in delivering that volume is the dependent variable, determined by the compliance of the lung and chest wall. The major advantage of this type of ventilator is the known, fixed tidal volume (V_T). Hence the $\dot{V}_E$ can be predictably set. Virtually all volume-cycled ventilators have pressure monitors and alarms to alert the medical staff if the pressure required to deliver the desired volume reaches dangerous levels, as may occur with falling lung compliance.

Time-Cycled Ventilator

The time-cycled ventilator also delivers a volume of air under positive pressure. However in this case, the flow ($\dot{V}$) and the time (t) for delivering each breath are the controlled factors. The subsequent volume delivered is simply calculated:

$$\dot{V} = V_T/t$$

$$V_T = \dot{V} \times t$$

Hence the time-cycled ventilator also allows direct control of the volume delivered as well as the $\dot{V}_E$. Like the volume-cycled ventilator, the pressure required to generate this flow within the designated time will vary with the lung and chest wall compliance. Pressure monitors and alarms are also an important part of these machines. The major advantages of the time-cycled over the volume-cycled ventilators are their small size and quiet operation. They also allow greater flexibility in adjusting the stream of inflation.

High-Frequency Ventilators

High-frequency ventilation is a different type of mechanical ventilation. With these machines, ventilation does not attempt to reproduce normal patterns of breathing; they do not deliver a tidal volume (V_T) of air at a normal respiratory frequency (F). Instead, very small volumes of air are injected or oscillated at frequencies ranging from 60 to 3000 cycles/min in the upper airway through the tracheal tube. The frequency and/or the volume may be controlled.

High-frequency ventilation probably provides air for gas exchange by facilitating diffusion and mixing of the gas within the tracheobronchial tree. The three common methods used for high-frequency ventilation are

- *High-frequency positive-pressure ventilation* (F = 60–120 cycles/min; V_T = 3–5 ml/kg body weight)
- *High-frequency jet ventilation* (F = up to 400 cycles/min; V_T = 2–5 ml/kg body weight)
- *High-frequency oscillation* (F = up to 3000 cycles/min; V_T = up to 3 ml/kg body weight)

The use of these ventilators remains controversial. However, high-frequency ventilation may play a particular role in patients who require ventilatory support but need a low mean airway pressure to permit healing of a bronchopleural fistula or a flail chest. Conventional methods should still be tried first.

INITIATING MECHANICAL VENTILATION

Any of the ventilators listed in the previous section is capable of adequately ventilating most patients, if managed properly. The goal of mechanical ventilation is adequate gas exchange. Achievement of this goal can only be measured with an ABG. Following are the steps for the initial management of a patient receiving mechanical ventilation.

- The *initial settings* are determined by estimating the patient's needs from knowledge of his basic respiratory and metabolic problems.
- *Check an ABG* to determine the adequacy of these initial settings in achieving the desired gas exchange.
- *Adjust the initial ventilator settings* to correct for deficiencies in the measured ABG.
- Each time the ventilator settings are adjusted, a *follow-up ABG* must be measured to see the effect of the change.

Selecting Initial Ventilator Settings

Table 1 lists guidelines for the initial ventilator settings, using a volume-cycled ventilator. These are empiric criteria that may not be appropriate for all patient situations. Clinical evaluation of the patient must come first, and the patient must be observed carefully in order to synchronize him with the ventilator. The patient ventilator system should be consistent with spontaneous respiration. Tidal volume settings (normally 10–13 ml/kg body weight) may need to be reduced if the patient has reduced lung volumes (from restrictive lung disease or following lung resection). Lower respiratory rates are needed when patients have obstruc-

TABLE 1. Initial Ventilator Settings for Adults

Setting[a]	Value
V_T	10–13 ml/kg
F	10–30/min
F_{IO_2}	Room air—1.0
I:E ratio	1:2–3
Inspiratory hold	Adjust to I:E
Expiratory retard	Adjust to I:E
Sensitivity	Adjust to patient comfort, I:E, ABG
Peak flow	Adjust to I:E, peak pressure
Minute ventilation	5–15 liters/min
Mode	Assist–control

[a] V_T = tidal volume; F = respiratory frequency; F_{IO_2} = fraction of inspired oxygen; I:E ratio = inspiratory time to expiratory time ratio.

tive airway diseases, while higher rates may be used in patients with restrictive disease. The assist–control mode is selected to allow adequate ventilation with minimum patient effort. The I:E ratio recorded by the ventilator may be inaccurate in measuring the ratio of inspiration to expiration in patients with bronchospasm.

Adjusting the Initial Ventilator Settings

After initiating ventilation as outlined, the following factors must be evaluated and monitored to assess the adequacy of these settings:

- Peak and plateau airway pressures
- Exhaled volume
- ABG
- Systemic blood pressure and pulse

Peak and Plateau Airway Pressures. Although the patient should not experience apneic intervals (inspiration should directly follow expiration), the breaths must not follow so closely that expiration is incomplete and functional residual capacity progressively increases with each breath. This phenomenon, called *stacking,* steadily blows the lungs up larger with each breath, causing higher and higher airway pressures in the volume-cycled ventilator. It can be detected by noting an increasing peak pressure on the ventilator manometer. (Peak pressure is the highest pressure recorded on the ventilator manometer.) This rising peak pressure returns to a low level after the patient has been disconnected from the ventilator for a few seconds; on reconnection, the stepwise increase in peak pressure recurs. This is also associated with finding the exhaled volume to be less than V_T. It may be corrected by increasing the peak *flow* of each inflation or changing the waveform of the inflation, measures aimed at delivering each volume earlier in the cycle and quicker; the F and occasionally the V_T may also need to be reduced.

If the plateau airway pressures are consistently very high, the patient often has stiff, noncompliant lungs, requiring ventilation with higher F and lower V_T. Often, decreasing compliance is due to passive congestion of the lungs, with fluid overload, which may improve with diuresis. However, it may also portend oxygen toxicity, pneumonia, or progressive adult respiratory distress syndrome.

The peak airway pressure may also be very high because the patient is not well synchronized with the machine and is trying to exhale when the machine is inflating his lungs. This problem can be detected by observing the abdominal respiratory excursions and the general level of relaxation of the patient. When the problem of poor synchronization does occur, efforts must be made to calm the patient by talking to him and explaining the process while adjusting the rate and tidal volume to levels with which he is more comfortable. Occasionally mild sedation must be used. In patients who are delerious or beyond reason, occasionally ventilator synchronization can only be achieved by using paralyzing muscle relaxants (succinylcholine or pancuronium) combined with major sedation (morphine). This adjunctive therapy should be avoided unless absolutely necessary because it transfers the patient's life totally and instantaneously into the hands of hospital personnel and machines.

High peak pressures (above 50 cm H_2O) are undesirable because they increase the risk of intrathoracic barotrauma and they diminish venous return to the heart. See Complications of Mechanical Ventilation.

Exhaled Volume. The exhaled volume should equal V_T (excluding 50–100 ml allowed for a cuff leak). In pressure-cycled ventilators, the exhaled volume is the only measurement of V_T; these ventilators must be adjusted so that this exhaled V_T multiplied by the respiratory F gives the desired $\dot{V}_E$ and $\dot{V}_A$. In the volume- and time-cycled ventilators, when the exhaled volume is less than the V_T, there is either a leak in the system (machine, tubing, tracheal tube, or balloon cuff) or the patient (bronchopleural or bronchocutaneous fistula), or the phenomenon of stacking described previously is occurring; the latter is confirmed by noting a stepwise increase in peak pressure.

However, finding the inspiratory volume equal to the expiratory volume does not guarantee that the patient has received all of this volume. Although the tubing connecting the patient to the ventilator is stiff, nevertheless, some volume can be lost during inflation in the stretching of this tubing; this volume is recovered and measured during exhalation although it never reached the lung. (See Fig. 1.) As a general rule, the less compliant the lungs and chest wall and the longer the tubing, the greater is the fraction of volume lost in the tubing. F may need to be increased to compensate for this problem.

Arterial Blood Gases. Although the measurements of pressure and volume are important factors in synchronizing the ventilator with the mechanics of the patient's natural respiratory apparatus, the ABG measurement is even more important in order to know the success of gas exchange. The mechanical measurements may look fine while the gas exchange remains poor. No clinical factors substitute for the measurement of the ABG.

Persistent, severe *hypoxemia* on the ABG obtained after initial settings requires an increase in oxygen delivery to the gas-exchanging units. This can be achieved by

- Increasing $\dot{V}_A$ (F or V_T)
- Increasing F_{IO_2}
- Adding positive end-expiratory pressure (PEEP, discussed below)

When the lungs are stiff and pressures mitigate against increasing V_T, the

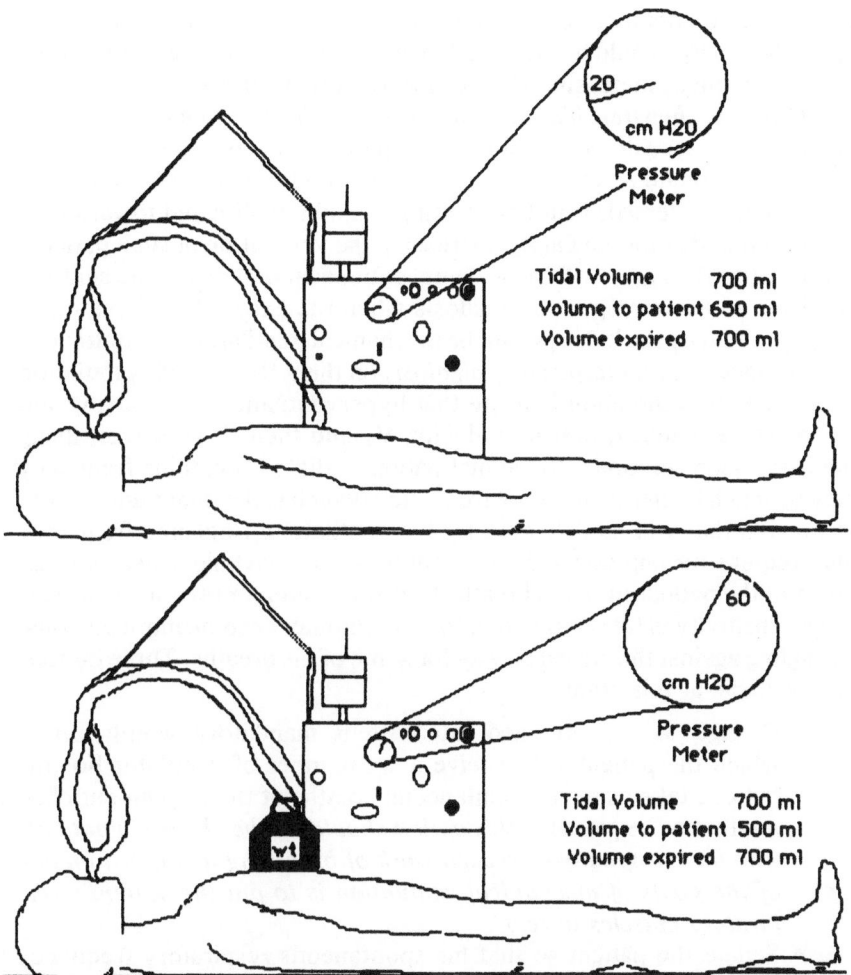

FIGURE 1. A decrease in lung compliance (as measured by an increase in peak/plateau pressure from 20 to 60 cm H_2O) will result in further loss of the "set" tidal volume (700 cc) in additional tubing expansion; however, this volume will be returned during expiration.

FI_{O_2} may be increased. However, sustained high concentrations of oxygen above 0.40, carry a risk of oxygen-induced lung injury. Furthermore, when the primary pulmonary problem involves right-to-left shunting (as in pneumonia, pulmonary edema, or adult respiratory distress syndrome), increasing the FI_{O_2} does little to improve the Pa_{O_2}. In these cases, the addition of PEEP may be required. (See PEEP.)

Hypercarbia on the ABG following initiation of mechanical ventilation may indicate that the $\dot{V}_A$ is still inadequate. However, it must be considered in conjunction with the pH. If acidosis accompanies the elevated Pa_{CO_2}, $\dot{V}_E$ should be increased by increasing V_T or, if peak pressures are already high, increasing F, in order to increase the $\dot{V}_A$.

However, *hypercarbia with a normal or high pH,* often indicates that the patient is accustomed to chronic respiratory acidosis and has a high serum bicarbonate level. Unless the chronic underlying problem can be substantially reversed, ventilator settings should be directed toward normalizing the pH, not the Pa_{CO_2}. Increasing the ventilation of such patients to normalize the Pa_{CO_2} will cause complications: at first metabolic acidosis and later an acute respiratory acidosis when the excess bicarbonate has been excreted by the kidneys and the mechanical ventilation discontinued.

Hypocarbia and respiratory alkalosis on the ABG following initiation of mechanical ventilation indicate that hyperventilation is occurring and $\dot{V}E$ must be reduced, first by reducing V_T and then F. However, using the assist–control mode, the actual patient-initiated breathing frequency may be much higher than the set frequency (which is the minimum number of breaths that will be delivered by the ventilator). Reducing frequency may require turning down the sensitivity of the machine sensor so that fewer of the patient-initiated breaths trigger a ventilator breath. However, if the sensitivity is turned too low, the patient may become more anxious, struggling against the closed airway for some of his breaths. Three options are available at this point.

- Change to synchronized intermittent mandatory ventilation in which the patient will receive a set number of ventilator breaths but can take as many spontaneous breaths of the oxygen-enriched mixture as he pleases. *This option should not be chosen in patients who have a greatly increased work of breathing and in whom one of the goals of mechanical ventilation is to put the patient's respiratory muscles to rest.*
- Sedate the patient so that his spontaneous respiratory frequency decreases and the F can be more easily controlled.
- Add dead space tubing to the endotracheal tube so that a larger part of each breath never reaches the gas-exchanging units. This method should not be used in patients who have substantial trouble with oxygenation, because it decreases $\dot{V}_A$.

Blood Pressure. A significant fall in the patient's systemic blood pressure on the initial ventilator settings may be due to a reduction in venous return and hence cardiac output caused by the positive intrathoracic pressure generated by the ventilator. When this occurs, make certain that the patient's intravascular fluid volume is adequate. Simple infusion of i.v. fluids may solve this problem. However, there may be concomitant cardiac impairment, requiring a reduction in ventilatory pressures; this can be done by reducing V_T and increasing F to maintain an adequate $\dot{V}_E$. The use of PEEP in this setting must be guarded because it may further reduce cardiac output.

Positive End-Expiratory Pressure

Positive end-expiratory pressure (PEEP) can be added to most positive pressure ventilators. It works by increasing the functional residual capacity of the patient, holding open (by positive pressure) small airways and alveoli throughout the entire respiratory cycle to provide a longer time for gases to diffuse across the alveolar–capillary surface.

PEEP should be considered for patients in whom the F_{IO_2} has been raised to or above 0.6 in order to maintain the Pa_{O_2} between 55 and 60 mm Hg. Although PEEP can be used in several situations, its main use is in patients with the respiratory distress syndrome.

The level of PEEP used varies from 5 to 20 cm H_2O; higher levels are occasionally used but carry a significant risk of causing barotrauma and depression of cardiac output. (See next section.) By applying continuous positive pressure throughout expiration, pulmonary capillary blood flow may be impaired, reducing venous return to the heart and diminishing cardiac output. Hence, although the Pa_{O_2} may improve with PEEP, if the cardiac output falls, oxygen transport will decline, reducing overall tissue oxygenation, which is antithetical to the ultimate goal of ventilation. The level of PEEP must be chosen that will balance improvement in the Pa_{O_2} with maintenance of an adequate cardiac output ($\dot{Q}$). (See Fig. 2.) Various criteria for finding the optimal level of PEEP are given in Table 2. Measuring compliance (using the ventilator's pressure manometer) is usually an excellent noninvasive method of following the effect of increasing levels of PEEP on the venous return and hence cardiac output. With increasing levels of PEEP, falling compliance correlates with a falling cardiac output. However, overall tissue oxygenation is best assessed by measuring the $P\bar{v}_{O_2}$ or $S\bar{v}_{O_2}$ in blood obtained from the pulmonary artery. In the appropriate patient, PEEP levels should be increased until either the Pa_{O_2} rises to 60 mm Hg (with an F_{IO_2} less than

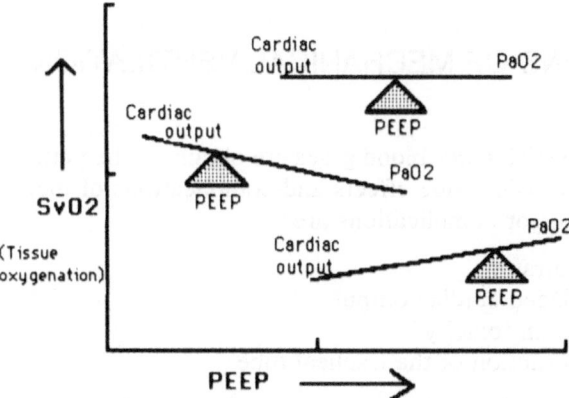

FIGURE 2. Influence of PEEP on tissue oxygenation ($S\bar{v}_{O_2}$). See text for discussion.

TABLE 2. Determining the Optimal Level of PEEP

Goals	Measurement	Comments
*1. Pa_{O_2} 60–70, Sa_{O_2} 0.90[a]	ABG	This Pa_{O_2} gives satisfactory O_2 content if Hb is normal
2. $F_{I_{O_2}} < 0.60$	Ventilator setting	This minimizes O_2 toxicity
3. PEEP as low as possible to achieve goals above and below	Ventilator setting	To minimize barotrauma and maximize venous return
**4. Compliance as high as possible[a]	Vt/plateau pressure	Best noninvasive means of estimating venous return and the effect of PEEP on cardiac output (with increasing PEEP, falling compliance correlates with falling venous return)
5. Cardiac output as high as possible	Right-heart catheterization— thermal or dye dilution technique	To maximize oxygen transport
***6. $P\bar{v}_{O_2} > 35$ mm Hg, $S\bar{v}_{O_2}$ 0.65–0.70[a]	Right-heart catheterization— pulmonary artery blood sample	Best overall means of assessing tissue oxygenation

[a] Asterisks indicate key parameters for determining optimal PEEP, in ascending order of importance. * = 1; ** = 2; *** = 3.

or equal to 0.60), or the lung compliance, cardiac output, or $S\bar{v}_{O_2}$ begins to fall.

COMPLICATIONS OF MECHANICAL VENTILATION

Once satisfactory blood gases are obtained, the patient must be monitored for possible side effects and complications of mechanical ventilation. The major complications are

- Barotrauma
- Reduced cardiac output
- Oxygen toxicity
- Obstruction of the tracheal tube

The manifestations, diagnosis, prevention, and treatment of these are summarized in Table 3.

TABLE 3. Complications of Mechanical Ventilation

	Manifestation	Cause	Prevention	Diagnosis	Treatment
Barotrauma Pneumothorax or mediastinum, subcutaneous emphysema	Chest pain Increasing pulse, and respiratory rate Decreasing Pa_{O_2} Swelling of face, neck, or chest	Increasing airway pressures cause air to rupture into the pleural space, mediastinum, or soft tissues of neck and abdomen	Keep peak and plateau airway pressures as low as possible	Auscultation of mediastinal crunch, unilateral absence of breath sounds Chest x ray Crepitations on physical examination	Pneumothorax requires a chest tube Lower the peak airway pressure May require high-frequency ventilation
Reduced cardiac output	Increasing pulse with falling blood pressure	Increased intrathoracic pressure obstructs venous return	Keep peak and plateau airway pressures as low as possible, monitor fluid status, and maintain hydration	Measure Pcwp, cardiac output, and/ or mixed venous O_2 tension, reassess parameters after lower airway pressure	Infuse i.v. fluids Reduce airway pressure (Vt) May need intra-aortic balloon pump
Oxygen toxicity	Decreasing Pa_{O_2} with increasing FI_{O_2}	Sustained (more than 48 hr) high oxygen concentrations (above 50%)	Keep FI_{O_2} to the lowest possible level, minimize O_2 requirements	ABG Chest x ray	Reduce FI_{O_2} if possible Glucocorticoids
Tracheal tube obstruction Secretions, blood, herniation of the balloon cuff	Increasing peak airway pressures May be stacking if there is a ball-valve effect	Secretions, blood, or herniation of the tube's balloon cuff	Regular tracheal tube care, frequent suctioning, monitoring of the cuff pressures	May require bronchoscopy for diagnosis	If suctioning is not successful, replace endotracheal or tracheostomy tube

Monitoring of the following factors will give an early warning of complications arising as well as indicating the patient's readiness for weaning:

Patient	Ventilator
Level of consciousness	Mode of ventilation
Spontaneous respiratory rate	Ventilator frequency
Heart rate	Tidal volume (V_T)
Blood pressure	Exhaled volume
Chest auscultation	Plateau airway pressure
Fluid intake/output	Peak airway pressure
Tracheal cuff pressure	F_{IO_2}
ABG	PEEP
Chest x ray	
P_IMAX	
Vital capacity	
Tidal volume	

In general, to minimize complications, fluid replacement must be kept adequate to maintain the cardiac output; the oxygen concentration of the inspired gas mixture must be kept as low as possible to maintain a Pa_{O_2} above 55–60 mm Hg (90% Sa_{O_2}), and peak airway pressures kept as low as possible while still providing adequate gas exchange. Occasionally it is necessary to further reduce oxygen requirements by reducing the patient's body temperature and muscle activity.

DISCONTINUING MECHANICAL VENTILATION

In many cases discontinuation of mechanical ventilation does not require weaning. The patient's capacity for spontaneous ventilation can be predicted from measurements taken while he is being ventilated. The measurements that predict a high likelihood of patient success with spontaneous ventilation are given in Table 4. However, even if the patient's measurements meet these criteria, mechanical ventilation should not be discontinued if the patient is in shock or has serious arrhythmias. Other relative contraindications to discontinuing mechanical ventilation in the face of satisfactory respiratory measurements include

- Poor nutritional status
- Acid–base imbalance
- Marked hypertension or a rapidly changing cardiovascular status,
- Presence of a progressive neuromuscular disorder.

The patient with severe chronic airflow obstruction (CAO) must be considered in a special category with regard to weaning criteria, because he may never meet the criteria listed in Table 4. In this patient, predicting

TABLE 4. Criteria for Discontinuing
Mechanical Ventilation

Minimal vital capacity—10–15 ml/kg

Minimal inspiratory force— >20 cm H_2O
(negative pressure)

Vd/Vt—<0.6

$P(A\text{-}a)_{O_2}$ on 100% O_2—<300–350 mm Hg

---

the ease and success of ventilator weaning is best done by observing the patient during a short trial off mechanical support.

When patients have been mechanically ventilated for a short interval of 1–4 days, have no or mild remaining respiratory dysfunction (easily meeting the criteria for weaning), and are otherwise stable, they can usually be taken directly off the ventilator and given supplemental oxygen to breathe through the tracheal tube at a slightly higher concentration than they were receiving on the ventilator. Most of these patients will remain stable (respiratory rate, heart rate, blood pressure, ABG) and be ready to be extubated within 30–60 min.

When patients have been ventilated for prolonged periods of time or continue to have significant respiratory impairment, progressive weaning techniques must be employed. Weaning is particularly difficult in patients with severe CAO. Although some clinicians prefer the use of successive reductions in the rate of intermittent mandatory ventilation for weaning, we find the use of successively longer periods on continuous positive airway pressure (CPAP), off the ventilator, to be more efficient. This method uses the following procedure:

1. Before weaning and periodically after, monitor the following:
   - Heart rate (rise of 20–30/min significant)
   - Blood pressure (BP) (rising BP warns of stress)
   - Spontaneous respiratory rate (RR) (rising RR suggests decreasing gas exchange)
   - Spontaneous tidal volume (decreasing V_T suggests respiratory muscle fatigue)
   - Spontaneous minute ventilation (increasing $\dot{V}_E$ suggests hypoxemia or acidosis, falling level may signify respiratory failure)
   - ABG (rise in Pa_{CO_2} and fall in Pa_{O_2} signify respiratory failure)
   - Thoracoabdominal coordination (discoordinate thoracoabdominal movement is a particularly useful sign of respiratory failure in CAO)
2. Transfer the patient from positive-pressure ventilation to CPAP with a slightly increased F_{IO_2} and monitor the above noninvasive measurements at intervals of 5 min or less. Check the ABG every 15 min for the first hour, then hourly or immediately before returning the patient to the mechanical ventilator to rest.

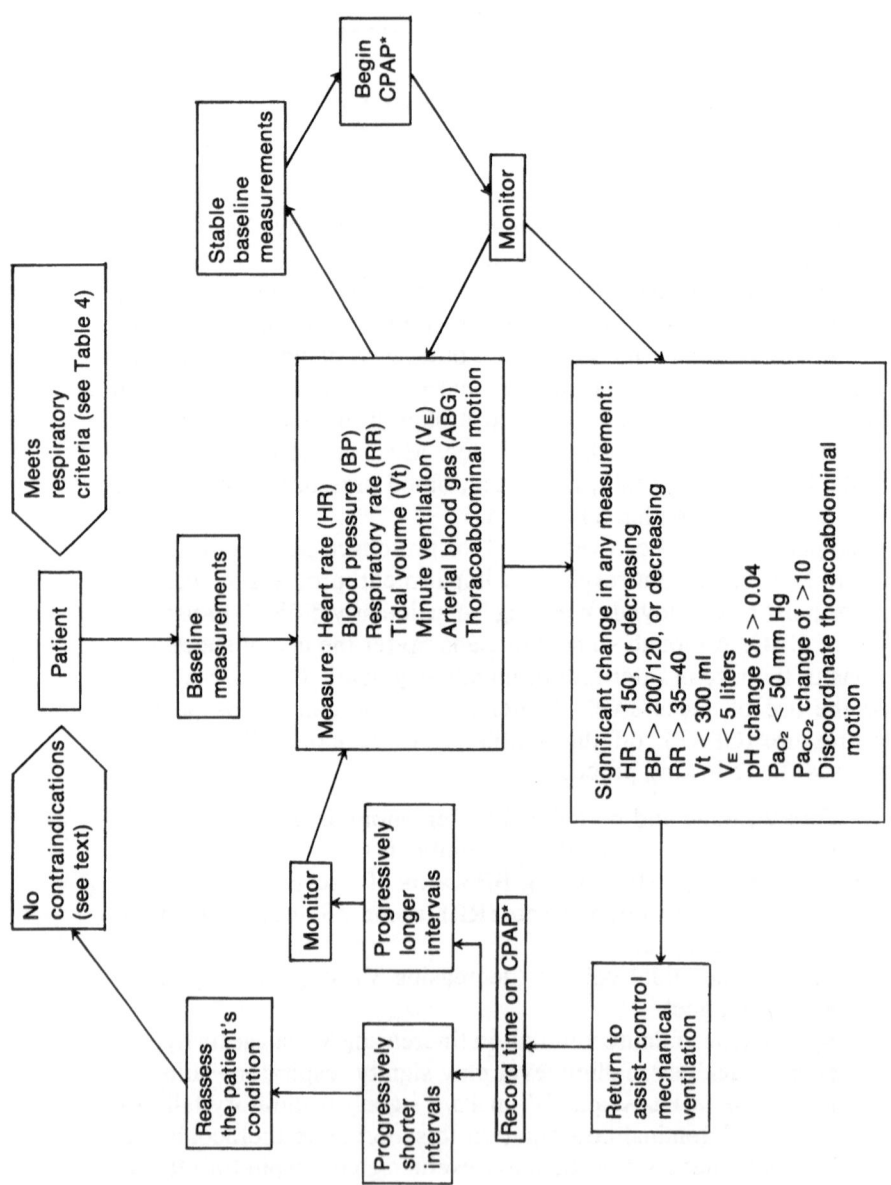

FIGURE 3. Discontinuing mechanical ventilation. *, See text for discussion.

3. When any of these measurements changes significantly from the baseline values, obtain an ABG and return the patient to mechanical ventilation on the assist–control mode; record the time he spent on CPAP.
4. Repeat the measurements listed in step 1 after 20 min back on the ventilator and monitor the noninvasive measurements until they are stable again.
5. Once the patient's measurements have returned to his baseline, and he has rested, transfer him back to CPAP with the increased F_{IO_2}.
6. Resume the periodic measurements and proceed according to steps 2–5 above.

Using this method, the patient usually doubles his time off the ventilator with each successive trial. If his time off decreases with successive trials, he may not be ready for weaning; reevaluate the patient for contraindications to weaning, listed above. Patients may be rested on the ventilator after a prolonged trial off, or overnight, this allows adequate time for sleep when the weaning process is protracted. This method has the advantage of progressive training of the respiratory muscles, allowing the patient complete rest of his respiratory muscles on the assist–control mode of the mechanical ventilator between trials. For this reason it is especially useful in working with patients who have severe CAO. However, it does require intensive nursing supervision. This method is summarized in Fig. 3.

CONCLUSION

Mechanical ventilation may be the most lifesaving therapeutic modality in patients with ventilatory failure. This chapter has reviewed principles of mechanical ventilation, types of ventilators available and their advantages, airway considerations, methods for initiating, adjusting, and discontinuing mechanical ventilation, and complications that arise from this form of treatment.

BIBLIOGRAPHY

1. Feeley TW, Hedley-Whyte J: Weaning from controlled ventilation and supplemental oxygen. *N Engl J Med* 292:903–906, 1975.
2. Jenkinson SG: Nutritional problems during mechanical ventilation in acute respiratory failure. *Respir Care* 28:641–645, 1983.

3. Morganroth ML, Morganroth JL, Nett LM, et al: Criteria for weaning from prolonged mechanical ventilation. *Arch Intern Med* 144:1012–1016, 1984.
4, Pierson DJ: Indications for mechanical ventilation in acute respiratory failure. *Respir Care* 28:570–578, 1983.
5. Petty TL: Intermittent mandatory ventilation—reconsidered. *Crit Care Med* 9:620–621, 1981.
6. Zwillich CW, Pierson DJ, Creagh CE, et al: Complications of assisted ventilation. *Am J Med* 57:161–170, 1974.

Terms and Symbols*

TERMS AND SYMBOLS

A. General symbols

1. P	Pressure, blood or gas
2. $\bar{X}$	A mean value, indicated by a dash over the symbol
3. $\dot{X}$	A time derivative indicated by a dot above the symbol (rate). This symbol is used for both instantaneous flow and volume per unit time
4. %X	Percent sign preceding a symbol indicates percentage of the predicted normal value
5. X/Y%	Percent sign following a symbol indicates a ratio function with the ratio expressed as a percentage. Both components of the ratio must be designated; e.g., $FEV_1/FVC\% = 100 \times FEV_1/FVC$
6. XA or Xa	A small capital letter or lower case letter on the same line following a primary symbol is a qualifier to further define the primary symbol. When small capital letters are not available on typewriters or to printers, large capital letters may be used as subscripts; e.g., $X_A = XA$

B. Gas phase symbols

1. Primary symbols (large capital letters)

a. V	Gas volume. The particular gas as well as its pressure, water vapor conditions, and other special conditions must be specified in text or indicated by appropriate qualifying symbols
b. F	Fractional concentration of a gas

* Report of the ACCP-ATS Joint Committee on Pulmonary Nomenclature: Pulmonary terms and symbols. *Chest* 67:583–593, 1975.

2. Common qualifying symbols
   a. I   Inspired
   b. E   Expired
   c. A   Alveolar
   d. T   Tidal
   e. D   Dead space or wasted ventilation
   f. B   Barometric
   g. L   Lung
   h. STPD   Standard conditions: Temperature 0°C, pressure 760 mm Hg and dry (0 water vapor)
   i. BTPS   Body conditions: Body temperature, ambient pressure, and saturated with water vapor at these conditions
   j. f   Respiratory frequency per minute
   k. max   Maximal
   l. est   Estimated
   m. t   Time

C. Blood phase symbols
   1. Primary symbols (large capital letters)
      a. Q   Blood volume
      b. Q̇   Blood flow, volume units, and time must be specified
      c. C   Concentration in the blood phase
      d. S   Saturation in the blood phase
   2. Qualifying symbols (lower-case letters)
      a. b   Blood in general
      b. a   Arterial
      c. c   Capillary
      d. c̀   Pulmonary end-capillary
      e. v   Venous
      f. v̄   Mixed venous

D. Ventilation and lung mechanics tests and symbols
   1. Lung volume compartments (Primary compartments are designated as volumes. When volumes are combined they are designated as capacities. All are considered to be at BTPS unless otherwise specified.)
      a. RV   Residual volume; that volume of air remaining in the lungs after maximal exhalation. The method of measurement should be indicated in the text or, when necessary, by appropriate qualifying symbols
      b. ERV   Expiratory reserve volume; the maximal volume of air exhaled from the end-expiratory level
      c. TV   Tidal volume; that volume of air inhaled or exhaled with each breath during quiet breathing, used only to indicate a subdivision of lung vol-

ume. When lung volume is used in gas exchange formulations, the symbol Vt should be used

d. IRV   Inspiratory reserve volume; the maximal volume of air inhaled from the end-inspiratory level

e. IC   Inspiratory capacity; the sum of IRV and TV

f. VC   Vital capacity; the maximum volume of air exhaled from the point of maximum inspiration

g. FRC   Functional residual capacity; the sum of RV and ERV (the volume of air remaining in the lungs at the end-expiratory position). The method of measurement should be indicated as with RV

h. TLC   Total lung capacity; the sum of all volume compartments or the volume of air in the lungs after maximal inspiration. The method of measurement should be indicated, as with RV

i. RV/TLC%   Residual volume to total lung capacity ratio, expressed as a percent

j. CV   Closing volume; the volume exhaled after the expired gas concentration is inflected from an alveolar plateau during a controlled breathing maneuver. Since the value obtained is dependent on the specific test technique, the method used must be designated in the text and, when necessary, specified by a qualifying symbol. Closing volume is often expressed as a ratio of the VC, i.e., CV/VC%

k. CC   Closing capacity; closing volume plus residual volume, often expressed as a ratio of TLC, i.e., CC/TLC%

l. VL   Actual volume of the lung, including the volume of the conducting airways

m. VA   Alveolar gas volume

2. Forced spirometry measurements (All values are BTPS unless otherwise specified.)

a. FVC   Forced vital capacity; vital capacity performed with a maximally forced expiratory effort

b. FIVC   Forced inspiratory vital capacity; the maximal volume of air inspired with a maximally forced effort from a position of maximal expiration

c. FEVt   Forced expiratory volume (timed). The volume of air exhaled in the specified time during the performance of the forced vital capacity; eg, FEV_1 for the volume of air exhaled during the first second of the FVC

d. FEVt/FVC%   Forced expiratory volume (timed) to forced vital capacity ratio, expressed as a percentage

e. FEFx   Forced expiratory flow, related to some portion of the FVC curve. Modifiers refer to the amount of the FVC already exhaled when the measurement is made

   FEF25–75%   Mean forced expiratory flow during the middle half of the FVC (formerly called the maximum mid-expiratory flow rate)

f. PEF   The highest forced expiratory flow measured with a peak flow meter

g. $\dot{V}$maxX   Forced expiratory flow, related to the total lung capacity of the actual volume of the lung at which the measurement is made. Modifiers refer to the amount of lung volume remaining when the measurement is made. For example: Vmax75% = instantaneous forced expiratory flow when the lung is at 75% of its TLC. $\dot{V}$max3.0 = instantaneous forced expiratory flow when the lung volume is 3.0 liters

h. MVVx   Maximal voluntary ventilation. The volume of air expired in a specified period during repetitive maximal respiratory frequency is indicated by a numerical qualifier; e.g., MVV60 is MVV performed at 60 breaths/min. If no qualifier is given, an unrestricted frequency is assumed

i. FIFx   Forced inspiratory flow. As in the case of the FEF, the appropriate modifiers must be used to designate the volume at which flow is being measured. Unless otherwise specified, the volume qualifiers indicate the volume inspired from RV at the point of the measurement

3. Measurements of ventilation (Unless otherwise specified, conditions are as indicated in parentheses.)

a. $\dot{V}$e   Expired volume per minute (BTPS)
b. $\dot{V}$I   Inspired volume per minute (BTPS)
c. $\dot{V}CO_2$ Carbon dioxide production per minute (STPD)
d. $\dot{V}O_2$ Oxygen consumption per minute (STPD)
e. $\dot{V}$A   Alveolar ventilation per minute (BTPS)
   VtA   Alveolar tidal volume (BTPS)
f. $\dot{V}$d   Ventilation per minute of the physiologic dead space (wasted ventilation), BTPS, defined by the following equation:

$$\dot{V}d = \dot{V}e(Pa_{CO_2}-Pe_{CO_2})/(Pa_{CO_2}-Pi_{CO_2})$$

  g. Vd   The physiologic dead-space volume defined as: $\dot{V}d/f$

4. Measurements of mechanics of breathing (All pressures are expressed relative to ambient pressure and gases are at BTPS unless otherwise specified.)

  a. Pressure terms

    Paw   Pressure in the airway, level to be specified
    Ppl   Intrapleural pressure
    Pa   Alveolar pressure
    Pl   Transpulmonary pressure
    Pes   Esophageal pressure used to estimate Ppl

  b. Flow pressure relationships (Unless otherwise specified, the lung volume at which all resistance measurements are made is assumed to be FRC.)

    R   A general symbol for resistance, pressure per unit flow
    Raw   Airway resistance
    Rl   Total pulmonary resistance, measured by relating flow-dependent transpulmonary pressure to airflow at the mouth
    Gaw   Airway conductance, the reciprocal of Raw
    Gaw/Vl   Specific conductance, expressed per liter of lung volume at which G is measured

  c. Volume–pressure relationships

    C   A general symbol for compliance, volume change per unit of applied pressure
    Cst   Static compliance, compliance determined from measurements made during conditions of prolonged interruption of air flow
    W   A general symbol for mechanical work of breathing, which requires use of appropriate qualifying symbols and description of specific conditions

E. Diffusing capacity tests and symbols

  1. Dx   Diffusing capacity of the lung expressed as volume (STPD) of gas (X) intake per unit alveolar-capillary pressure difference for the gas used. Unless otherwise stated, carbon monoxide is assumed to be the test gas: i.e., D is Dco. A modifier can be used to designate the technique: e.g., Dsb is single-breath carbon monoxide-diffusing capacity and Dss is steady-state CO-diffusing capacity

  2. Dm   Diffusing capacity of alveolar capillary membrane (STPD)

F. Blood gas measurements

Symbols for these values are readily composed by combining the general symbols recommended earlier. Some examples include:

1. Pa_{CO_2} Arterial carbon dioxide tension
2. Sa_{O_2} Arterial oxygen saturation
3. Cc_{O_2} Oxygen content of pulmonary end-capillary blood
4. $P(A-a)_{O_2}$ Alveolar–arterial oxygen pressure difference. The previously used symbol, $A-aD_{O_2}$ is not recommended.
5. $C(a-v)_{O_2}$ Arteriovenous oxygen content difference

G. Pulmonary shunts

1. $\dot{Q}sp$ Physiologic shunt flow (total venous admixture) defined by the following equation when gas and blood data are collected during ambient air breathing:

$$\dot{Q}sp = \frac{Cc_{O_2} - Ca_{O_2}}{Cc_{O_2} - C\bar{v}_{O_2}} \times \dot{Q}$$

2. $\dot{Q}san$ A special case of $\dot{Q}sp$ (often called anatomic shunt flow) defined by the above equation when blood and gas data are collected after sufficiently prolonged breathing of 100% O_2 to assure an alveolar N_2 less than 1%. It can be estimated conveniently with the following equation:

$$\dot{Q}san = \frac{0.0031P(A-a)_{O_2}}{0.0031P(A-a)_{O_2} + C(a-\bar{v})_{O_2}} \times \dot{Q}$$

H. Pulmonary dysfunction

1. Terms related to altered breathing: There are many terms in use, such as tachypnea, hyperpnea, hypopnea. Simple descriptive terms, such as rapid, deep, or shallow breathing, should be used instead.

   a. Dyspnea: A subjective sensation of difficult or labored breathing.

   b. Overventilation: A general term indicating excessive ventilation. When unqualified, it refers to alveolar overventilation, excessive ventilation of the gas-exchanging areas of the lung manifested by a fall in arterial CO_2 tension. The term total overventilation may be used when the minute volume is increased regardless of the alveolar ventilation. (When there is increased wasted ventilation, total overventilation may occur when alveolar ventilation is normal or decreased.)

c. Underventilation: A general term indicating reduced ventilation. When otherwise unqualified, it refers to alveolar underventilation, decreased effective alveolar ventilation manifested by an increase in arterial CO_2 tension. (Over- and underventilation are recommended in place of hyper- and hypoventilation to avoid confusion when the words are spoken.)

2. Terms describing blood gas findings
   a. Hypoxia: A term for reduced oxygenation
   b. Hypoxemia: A reduced blood oxygen content or tension
   c. Hypocarbia (hypocapnia): A reduced arterial carbon dioxide tension
   d. Hypercarbia (hypercapnia): An increased arterial carbon dioxide tension

3. Terms describing acid–base findings
   a. Acidemia: A pH less than normal; the value should always be given
   b. Alkalemia: A pH greater than normal; the value should always be given
   c. Hypobasemia: Blood bicarbonate level below normal
   d. Hyperbasemia: Blood bicarbonate level above normal
   e. Acidosis: A clinical term indicating disturbance that can lead to acidemia. It is usually indicated by hypobasemia when metabolic (nonrespiratory) in origin and by hypercarbia when respiratory in origin. There may or may not be accompanying acidemia. The term should always be qualified as metabolic (nonrespiratory) or respiratory
   f. Alkalosis: A clinical term indicating a disturbance that can lead to alkalemia. It usually is indicated by hyperbasemia when metabolic (nonrespiratory) in origin and by hypocarbia when respiratory in origin. There may or may not be accompanying alkalemia. The term should always be qualified as metabolic (nonrespiratory) or respiratory

4. Other terms
   a. Pulmonary insufficiency: Altered function of the lungs that produces clinical symptoms, usually including dyspnea
   b. Acute respiratory failure: Rapidly occurring hypoxemia or hypercarbia due to a disorder of the respiratory system. The duration of the illness and the values of arterial oxygen tension and arterial carbon dioxide tension used as criteria for this term should be given. The term acute ventilatory failure should be used only when the arterial carbon dioxide tension is increased. The term pulmonary failure has been used to indicate respiratory failure due specifically to disorders of the lungs
   c. Chronic respiratory failure: Chronic hypoxemia or hypercapnia due to a disorder of the respiratory system. The duration of the condition and the values of arterial oxygen tension and

arterial carbon dioxide tension used as criteria for this term should be given

d. Obstructive pattern (obstructive ventilatory defect): Slowing of air flow during forced ventilatory maneuvers

e. Restrictive pattern (restrictive ventilatory defect): Reduction of vital capacity not explainable by airflow obstruction

f. Small airway dysfunction: There are newly described tests that purport to test function of small airways (closing volume, frequency dependence of compliance, flow–volume curves). When isolated abnormalities of these tests are found, the term "small airway dysfunction" is appropriate

g. Impairment: A measurable degree of anatomic or functional abnormality that may or may not have clinical significance. Permanent impairment is that which persists after maximum medical rehabilitation has been achieved

Normal Values*

VENTILATION (BTPS)

Tidal volume, liters	0.50
Frequency, breaths/min	12
Minute volume, liters/min	6.00
Respiratory dead space, ml	150
Alveolar ventilation, liters/min	4.20

LUNG VOLUMES (BTPS)

Vital capacity (VC), liters	4.50
Residual volume (RV), liters	1.50
Functional residual capacity (FRC), liters	3.00
Total lung capacity (TLC), liters	6.00
Residual volume/total lung capacity × 100(RV/TLC%)	25

MECHANICS OF BREATHING

Maximal voluntary ventilation (MVV), liters/min	170

* Values vary according to age, height, sex, and position (seated versus supine).

Forced expiratory volume in 1s ($FEV_1/FVC\%$)	75
Forced expiratory volume in 3s ($FEV_3/FVC\%$)	97
Forced expiratory flow during middle half of $FVC(FEF_{25-75\%})$, liters/sec	4.7
Static compliance of the lungs (Cl_{st}), liters/cm H_2O	0.2
Compliance of lungs and thoracic cage, liters/cm H_2O	0.1
Airway resistance at FRC (R_{aw}), cm H_2O liters/sec	1.5
Pulmonary resistance at FRC, cm H_2O liters/sec	2.0
Maximal inspiratory pressure, mm Hg	75
Maximal expiratory pressure, mm Hg	120

OXYGENATION

Pa_{O_2}, mm Hg	100
PA_{O_2}, mm Hg	110
$P(A\text{-}a)_{O_2}$, mm Hg	<25
R, mm Hg	0.8
$P\bar{v}_{O_2}$, mm Hg	40
Pa_{CO_2}, mm Hg	40
Sa_{O_2}, %	97
$S\bar{v}_{O_2}$, %	75
$P(a\text{-}\bar{v})_{O_2}$, mm Hg	30–50
pH	7.40 ± 0.04
Hb, g/100 cc	15
Oxygen content of blood, cc/ml	20
Oxygen transport (resting), cc/min	1000
Oxygen consumption (resting), cc/min	250

HEMODYNAMIC PARAMETERS

Cardiac output (resting), liters/min	5
Systemic vascular resistance, dyne-sec/cm^5	800–1200
Cardiac ejection fraction (resting)	>0.5

Pulmonary artery pressure

Systolic, mm Hg	25
Diastolic, mm Hg	12
Mean, mm Hg	16
Pulmonary capillary wedge pressure, mm Hg (mean)	10
Central venous pressure, mm Hg	6

MISCELLANEOUS

White blood cell count: total	$4.5–11 \times 10^3$
Neutrophils	54–62%
Band forms	3–5%
Eosinophils	1–3%
Monocytes	0–5%
Lymphocytes	25–33%
Serum electrolytes	
Na^+, mmole/liter	136–146
K^+, mmole/liter	3.5–5
Cl^-, mmole/liter	98–106
HCO_3^-, mmole/liter	21–28
Ca^{2+}, mg/dl	8.4–10.2
PO_4^{3-}, mg/dl	3.0–4.5
Therapeutic drug levels: theophylline, μg/ml	8–20

Index

t indicates that material is discussed in a table.

•